How To Be a Nurse Assistant

Making a Difference in Long Term Care

AMY BENNETT COATS, M. ED.
AND
MARGARET CASEY-MEDERIOS, RN

ahca
American Health Care Association

This edition of How To Be a Nurse Assistant was made possible through the support of our educational partners, Gulf South Medical Supply, Inc. and Kendall.

Project Manager: Robert L. Cavanaugh
Developmental Editor: Tom Lochhaas
Design: Westbound Publications, Inc.
Cover Design: HZDG

Printed in the United States of America by Courier Printing.

American Health Care Association
1201 L St. NW
Washington DC 20005-4015
www.ahca.org

"Well meant protectiveness gradually undermines any autonomy."

Ellen Langer
Mindfulness

About the Authors

AMY BENNETT COATS

Amy Bennett Coats has over 20 years experience as a manager, analyst, and educator within the health care industry. For the past 15 years she has been involved in the development of conferences, seminars, training programs, and compliance manuals for assisted living and nursing home providers and their employees.

Amy has worked for the American Health Care Association, the Assisted Living Federation of America, The American National Red Cross, and American Medical International.

Amy first collaborated with Margaret Casey-Mederios on the development of a nurse assistant training series for The American National Red Cross, which was published in 1989. They also developed training materials for direct care workers in assisted living for the American Health Care Association.

Amy has a master's degree in education, with an emphasis in human resource development, from The George Washington University.

MARGARET CASEY-MEDERIOS

Margaret (Peggy) Casey-Mederios has been a Registered Nurse for over 20 years. Her experience has been largely in the development of training for nurses and nurse assistants in all health care settings. Since 1983 Peggy has been writing and implementing training materials for nurse assistants and home health aides. The primary focus of the material she has developed has always been the desire to teach caregivers how to balance the tasks of their jobs with the ability to care. Peggy believes this balance is necessary to ensure quality care while maintaining the resident's, client's or patient's quality of life.

As an employee of The American National Red Cross, Peggy was the primary nursing writer for the organization's nurse assistant training materials published in 1989, a joint effort with Beverly Enterprises. These materials were implemented in various locations throughout Beverly's nursing facilities along with a number of The American National Red Cross chapters. Peggy also participated in The American National Red Cross's first edition of Foundations For Caregiving, a book that focused on cross training caregivers for long term, home health, and acute care.

In 1992, the American Health Care Association selected Peggy to author their second edition of How To Be a Nurse Assistant. This opportunity allowed Peggy to apply all her knowledge and experience in training nurse assistants into a package of textbook, workbook, and instructor's manual, focused on long term care. The success of How To Be a Nurse Assistant led to an inservice series for long term care and assisted living facilities also published by the American Heath Care Association.

Contents

To The Student:

This workbook is designed to be used as a study guide to help you learn the material you are reading in *How To Be a Nurse Assistant.* Be sure to read the chapters in the textbook before trying to complete the exercises in this workbook.

The textbook and the workbook are closely linked, so it is important for you to refer to the textbook as you complete each exercise. Unless your instructor suggests a different approach, work through the chapters in the workbook shortly after reading the matching chapter in the textbook. Answers to the exercises are in the Instructor's Manual.

A variety of exercises have been included in this workbook with the goal of appealing to your individual learning style. Formats include:

Crossword Puzzle
Essay
Fill in the Blank
Labeling
Matching
Multiple Choice
Spell It Out
True/False

Initial activities in each chapter, such as crossword puzzles, fill in the blank, matching, and spell it out, will call upon your ability to find, recall, and be familiar with medical and key terms. True/False, multiple-choice, and essay questions will help you to grasp concepts, relationships and rules. Labeling activities encourage you to recognize and relate pictures to words. Additional matching activities encourage you to think critically and decide how to handle realistic situations a nurse assistant will face. You will have the opportunity to prioritize activities, choose how to react to a difficult situation, or decide what to say to a resident or family member at an awkward moment.

Take the practice exam, found on pages 125-129, to help you prepare for the written portion of the state competency test. The procedure checklists beginning on page 131 will help guide you through successful completion of all direct care procedures described in the textbook.

Remember that the activities in the workbook are not intended to "test" you but to support what you learn from the textbook and in class. Have fun with these exercises, remember to refer to the textbook when necessary, and ask your instructor for help with any questions you can't answer.

Completing these exercises will better prepare you for completion of the training, successful completion of the state competency exam, and for your role as a nurse assistant.

Chapter 1

WHERE YOU WORK: THE LONG TERM CARE FACILITY

ACTIVITY 1 – FILL IN THE BLANK

Using the medical terms below, complete each sentence.

Chronic illness
Impairment
Intravenous

Occupational therapist
Onset
Physical therapist

Recreation therapy
Restorative
Speech therapist

Subacute care

1. A(n) _____ works with residents to improve their ability to walk.

2. Residents who do not need to be in the hospital but are not ready to be at home need _____ .

3. A condition that does not have a cure, has a gradual onset, and lasts a long time is called a(n) _____ .

4. A person who works with residents to improve or maintain their fine motor skills is called a(n) _____ .

5. Residents who have difficulty talking may work with a(n) _____ .

6. The purpose of _____ is to help residents stay active.

7. Blindness is an example of a(n) _____ .

8. Medication or fluids given to a resident through a blood vessel are _____ .

9. A plan of care designed to help someone return to health is called _____ .

10. The time at which a person first develops a disease is referred to as the _____ of that disease.

ACTIVITY 2 – CROSSWORD PUZZLE

Complete the puzzle by using the correct key term from the list, according to the clues below.

Accredit
Admission
Convalescent
Disability
Discharge
Gerontology
Interdisciplinary
Linen
Optimal
Preferences
Premiums
Rehabilitative
Residential
Respite
Risk management
Significant other

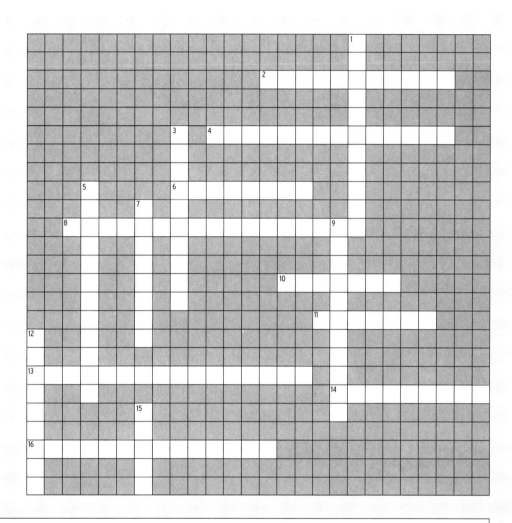

ACROSS

2. Personal choices or favorites

4. Restoring to former health

6. To recognize a facility that conforms to a standard

8. Involving 2 or more academic, scientific, or artistic disciplines

10. Most desirable or satisfactory

11. Interval of rest or relief

13. Person who is very close and important to another person (2 words)

14. Administrative procedure for entering a facility

16. Process of limiting legal liability (2 words)

DOWN

1. A branch of knowledge dealing with aging

3. Lack of a full physical or mental functioning

5. Recovering health and strength gradually after sickness or illness

7. Payments for insurance policies

9. Long term care facility where people live day and night

12. Administrative procedure for leaving a facility

15. Sheets, pillow cases, and mattress covers

ACTIVITY 3 – MULTIPLE CHOICE

Circle the letter beside the best answer.

1. Personal care activities do NOT include:
   A. Bathing
   B. Cooking
   C. Dressing
   D. Grooming

2. Subacute facilities provide specialized services for people who need:
   A. High levels of nursing care.
   B. Treatment for HIV or AIDs.
   C. Long term rehab for a head injury.
   D. Supervision so they won't wander.

3. People enter long term care facilities for:
   A. Rehabilitation.
   B. Supportive care.
   C. Many different reasons.
   D. High level nursing services.

4. What is the value of an interdisciplinary team approach to resident care?
   A. People enjoy being members of a team.
   B. One person doesn't have to do all the work.
   C. Information is shared and care is coordinated.
   D. Co-workers have a chance to chat with each other.

5. What does CMS stand for?
   A. Center for Medical Services
   B. Corporation for Medical Strategies
   C. Comprehensive Major Medical Supply
   D. Centers for Medicare and Medicaid Services

ACTIVITY 4 – TRUE/FALSE

In the space provided, write T for true or F for false.

1. _____ Everyone believes life is worth living as long as they have enough money.

2. _____ Life ends when a person enters long term care.

3. _____ The resident's care plan is used daily by the interdisciplinary team.

4. _____ The social worker is usually responsible for admitting a new resident.

5. _____ About half of all residents pay for long term care out of their savings.

6. _____ Medicaid pays for long term care costs for people with limited income.

7. _____ All long term care facilities provide dietary and pharmacy services.

8. _____ CMS requires long term care facilities to follow government rules and regulations.

9. _____ Long term care facilities are surveyed by the state every 5 years.

10. _____ All long term care facilities are accredited by JCAHO.

ACTIVITY 5 – IN YOUR OWN WORDS

1. Describe what makes life worth living for you.

2. Imagine what it must be like to live in a long term care facility. Describe how you would feel if you were a resident.

3. Make a list of things you would like to continue to do if you were a resident in a long term care facility.

STARTING YOUR JOB: WHAT TO EXPECT

ACTIVITY 1 – MATCHING

In the space provided, write the letter of the correct definition.

Term	Definition
1. _____ Ethics	A. To revive from apparent death
2. _____ Mindful	B. Involving 2 or more academic, scientific, or artistic disciplines
3. _____ Contracture	C. Separate section of a building attached to a central section
4. _____ Values	D. Continually being aware
5. _____ Culture	E. Beliefs people have about what is important to them
6. _____ Resuscitate	F. Designed to help a person return to health
7. _____ Interdisciplinary	G. A deformity caused by permanent shortening of a muscle or by scar tissue
8. _____ Restorative	H. Knowledge, awareness, or study of good and bad, right and wrong, and moral duty.
9. _____ Wing	I. The customary beliefs, social forms, and traits of a racial, social, or religious group

ACTIVITY 2 – TRUE/FALSE

Write T for True or F for False in the blank provided.

1. _____ A nurse assistant who provides care quickly is mindful.

2. _____ Our culture influences what foods we like, the clothes we wear, and how we worship.

3. _____ You gain a resident's trust by being reliable, respectful, caring, and honest.

4. _____ Nurse assistants are usually too busy to be concerned with residents' likes and dislikes.

5. _____ Mindful caregiving means making the effort to observe residents closely.

6. _____ Staffing shortages never affect caregiving in nursing facilities.

7. _____ For most people, stress is usually caused by financial concerns.

8. _____ The best way to cope with your emotions is to work through them on your own.

9. _____ An important way to get along with residents and co-workers is to respect their opinions and beliefs.

10. _____ Factors that influence care include break times and rainy days.

ACTIVITY 3 – MULTIPLE CHOICE

Circle the letter beside the best answer.

1. The term mindful caregiving means to:
   A. Provide care as quickly as possible.
   B. Give care in a thoughtful, efficient way.
   C. Always mind residents and their families.
   D. Spend an hour with each resident each day.

2. You balance the science of nursing with the art of caregiving when you:
   A. Find creative ways to get everything done.
   B. Make sure the resident's pants and shirt match.
   C. Pretend to listen to the resident as you give care.
   D. Talk with a resident as you give them a bed bath.

3. In order to have a good relationship with the charge nurse, you should:
   A. Offer to take her to lunch each week.
   B. Say nice things about her to all other staff.
   C. Be reliable, trustworthy, and communicate openly.
   D. Give her a present on her birthday and all major holidays.

4. A resident who is not assigned to you needs help toileting. You should:
   A. Tell them you are not their nurse assistant and walk away.
   B. Tell the resident to wait while you find their nurse assistant.
   C. Assist them with toileting then tell the other nurse assistant.
   D. Yell down the hall for the nurse assistant caring for that resident.

5. If you're not sure how to do an assignment, you should:
   A. Ask the housekeeper if she can help you.
   B. Talk to the charge nurse about your concerns.
   C. Do the best you can and hope it turns out O.K.
   D. Ask the resident how they think it should be done.

ACTIVITY 4 – MATCHING

Read each example and decide which term it reflects. Write the first letter of that term in the space provided. Refer to examples in the text-book if necessary.

Term

Culture   Ethics   Values

Example

1. _____ Mrs. DiCaprio has dressed in black every day since her husband died.

2. _____ Mr. Marlow's family has decided he should not be resuscitated if cardiac arrest happens.

3. _____ Mrs. Henderson always wants to look perfect before she leaves her room.

4. _____ Mr. Mooney doesn't want any special measures taken to keep him alive.

5. _____ Mrs. Logan reads the Bible every morning.

6. _____ Mrs. Anders was a volunteer for the Humane Society. She enjoys it when pets are brought into the facility.

7. _____ A member of Mrs. Nguyen's family brings her sushi at least once a week.

8. _____ You believe in providing the best care you can.

ACTIVITY 5 – YES OR NO

Read each example of caregiving. In the space provided, write YES if it is mindful caregiving, or NO if it is not.

1. _____ You listen to Mr. Morricone's preferences about his personal care and do exactly what he wants within safe limits.

2. _____ Mrs. Baker says she doesn't feel well today and doesn't want to walk. You tell her she needs to walk anyway.

3. _____ Mrs. Lawler is slow and confused today. You can't waste time, so you rush her along so that you can get to the next resident on your list.

4. _____ Mrs. Lim is very quiet today. You ask her if anything is bothering her.

5. _____ When you give Mr. Burrell his bath, you notice a red spot on his elbow. You report it to the charge nurse.

6. _____ Because you are running behind schedule, you pick Mrs. O'Hara's outfit instead of waiting for her to do so.

7. _____ As you help Mr. Quinn with his personal care, you ask him the latest news about his grandchildren.

8. _____ The daughter of a new resident is visiting today. You stop to talk with her and ask questions about her mother's preferences.

9. _____ Even though Mrs. Bradley says nothing is wrong, she seems flushed. You tell the charge nurse.

10. _____ Mr. Kayser asks you to find a newspaper for him just as your shift is ending. Without looking for one, you tell him they've all been thrown away.

ACTIVITY 6 — MATCHING

Next to each situation, write the letter of the correct response.

Situation	Response
1. _____ Mrs. Kelly complains that she is in pain. You think people should be able to live with a little pain.	A. Let the nurse assistant know, in a friendly way, that her voice is a little too loud.
2. _____ Mr. Daly's family has decided he should not have a feeding tube, even though he can no longer swallow. This decision is against your religious beliefs.	B. It would be wrong to impose your beliefs on the resident. Spiritual beliefs and practices are very personal.
3. _____ A resident never attends Sunday morning services, even though she is Christian. You think she needs spiritual guidance.	C. Don't let the family know you disapprove. Discuss you feelings with the charge nurse.
4. _____ A resident is asking you personal questions about her new roommate.	D. Put your own values aside. Ask the resident what hurts and tell the charge nurse promptly.
5. _____ Another nurse assistant on your shift talks so loudly residents have complained to you.	E. In a friendly way, bring up your concerns to the co-worker. Suggest that the 2 of you discuss work assignments with the charge nurse.
6. _____ Mrs. Greer believes Halloween is sinful and has criticized staff for making a big deal of it.	F. Remember that she is entitled to her beliefs. Respect her point of view.
7. _____ A co-worker has been asking for your help so often that you have to rush personal care for your own residents.	G. You explain that you aren't allowed to share personal information about any resident.

ACTIVITY 7 – IN YOUR OWN WORDS

In the space provided, describe why you think it is important to have a good relationship with the charge nurse and your co-workers.

Part A

The charge nurse can assist you to:

1.

2.

3.

4.

Part B

Your co-workers can assist you to:

1.

2.

3.

4.

ACTIVITY 8 – IN YOUR OWN WORDS

What kinds of questions should you ask the charge nurse when you get an assignment?

What can you do to develop a trusting relationship with your charge nurse?

Chapter 3

UNDERSTANDING EACH RESIDENT

ACTIVITY 1 – FILL IN THE BLANK

Using the correct medical or key term listed below, complete each sentence.

Amputation	Gross motor skills	Integrity	Reality	Theory
Assertive	Hierarchy	Need	Recognition	
Generativity	Imminent	Psychosocial	Status	

1. If something is necessary for life, it is a(n) _____ .

2. If something actually happened, it is a(n) _____ .

3. Abraham Maslow believed we all develop needs in a certain order, called _____ .

4. When scientists aren't able to explain something, they try to come up with a set of principles or ideas, called a(n) _____ .

5. If something is _____ , it is going to happen right away.

6. When we have accomplished something very important, we want _____ by our peers.

7. A person who behaves in a confident way is _____ .

8. If a middle-aged person feels they have created or accomplished something with their life, they have had success in experiencing _____ .

9. The ability to run, walk, or catch a ball involves the use of _____ _____ _____ .

10. If a resident receives respect and recognition from others, they have _____ .

11. A sense of feeling fulfilled, whole, or complete is called ego _____ .

12. A resident who has had an arm or leg cut off due to disease or injury has had a(n) _____ .

13. Issues that affect our mental and emotional health are called _____ issues.

ACTIVITY 2 – MULTIPLE CHOICE

Circle the letter beside the best answer.

1. Erickson believed the older adult needs to feel:
   A. They are still independent.
   B. They have lived successfully.
   C. They have created a work of art.
   D. They have made the world a good place.

2. Maslow believed that our higher level needs cannot be met:
   A. Unless all lower level needs are met.
   B. Unless we are living with our families.
   C. Until we have more food than we need.
   D. Until we have a lot of money in the bank.

3. You can help a resident meet their need for status by:
   A. Showing them respect.
   B. Changing their bed linens.
   C. Giving the resident a foot rub.
   D. Ensuring they eat a good breakfast.

4. A resident is being visited by their spouse and they want privacy. You should:
   A. Leave the door to the room open.
   B. Respect their desire to be alone together.
   C. Tell them they are not allowed to have sex.
   D. Report this information to the charge nurse.

5. We all have a basic need to:
   A. Remain independent.
   B. Achieve success at sports.
   C. Write the story of our life.
   D. Learn to speak another language.

ACTIVITY 3 – MATCHING

Match each basic need with an example in which that need is involved. Some needs will be used more than once.

Need

A. Physical
B. Safety and Security
C. Social
D. Status
E. Self-fulfillment

Example

1. _____ Responding to a resident who needs help getting to their bathroom.

2. _____ A resident shares photos from his many trips abroad with other residents.

3. _____ Seeing that a resident gets their dinner tray on time.

4. _____ A resident enjoying a visit with her great-grandchildren.

5. _____ Assisting the resident when they use the toilet.

6. _____ Wiping up a spill in the hallway of the facility.

7. _____ A resident knows that she will not be harmed in any way.

8. _____ A resident having a book of poetry published.

9. _____ Cutting meat for a resident with right-sided weakness.

10. _____ Helping a resident with grooming before a party.

ACTIVITY 4 – LABEL THE DIAGRAM

Using the list of needs in Activity 3, label each level of the pyramid. Remember that lower level needs are at the bottom.

1. _____

2. _____

3. _____

4. _____

5. _____

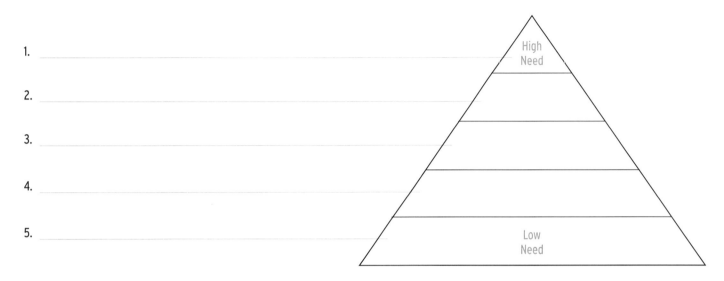

High Need

Low Need

ACTIVITY 5 – TRUE/FALSE

Write T for true or F for false in the space beside each statement.

1. _____ A resident who doesn't attend religious services does not have spiritual needs.

2. _____ A resident has less independence if you do everything for them.

3. _____ As a resident becomes more dependent on staff, they may have less self-worth.

4. _____ A frail or confused resident doesn't have sexual needs.

5. _____ A person's status needs must be met before they can meet their social needs.

6. _____ If a resident is in pain, their social needs become less important.

7. _____ Physical needs must be met before status needs become important.

8. _____ Knowing a resident well is the best way for you to meet their needs.

9. _____ Once a person has met a higher level need, they never have to worry about meeting a lower level need.

10. _____ How we feel about ourselves can depend on how others react to us.

1. What activities do you enjoy during your free time? How do these activities meet your needs?

_____

_____

_____

_____

2. Think about Maslow's hierarchy of needs. Give an example of an activity typical of how people meet each of the 5 levels of needs.

_____

_____

_____

_____

3. How can your understanding of different residents' needs assist you in giving care to residents? Give 3 specific examples.

_____

_____

_____

_____

4. List 2 ways you can assist residents in meeting their physical needs.

_____

_____

_____

_____

5. List 2 ways you can assist residents in meeting their status needs.

_____

_____

_____

_____

6. List 2 ways you can assist residents in meeting their sexual needs.

_____

_____

_____

_____

Chapter

UNDERSTANDING RESIDENTS' RIGHTS

In the space provided, write the letter of the correct definition.

Term	Definition
1. _____ Advocate	A. weakness
2. _____ Allegation	B. a person's statement or intended legal action
3. _____ At risk	C. someone who takes the side of another person and speaks for them.
4. _____ Battery	D. freedom to make your own choices and choose your own actions
5. _____ Confidentiality	E. keeping information private
6. _____ Frailty	F. retaliation against or punishment of a person for doing something
7. _____ Hearing	G. failure to do something that should have been done
8. _____ Incident	H. someone who has a probability of having some type of medical incident
9. _____ Neglect	I. move to another room in the facility
10. _____ Reprisal	J. a person's state or situation
11. _____ Right	K. something one has a just or legal claim to
12. _____ Securing	L. unlawful beating or use of force
13. _____ Self-determination	M. initial discussion of what happened when charges are made against someone
14. _____ Sentimental value	N. something happens that is unusual
15. _____ Status	O. making something safe
16. _____ Transfer	P. an object of value because of associations and memories it has for the owner

ACTIVITY 2 – FILL IN THE BLANK

Complete each sentence correctly, using the medical terms provided.

Chemical restraint
Circulation
Physical restraint
Sedate

1. Medication that is used to _____

   a resident or slow their muscle activity is called a

   _____   _____ .

2. Blood flows through our bodies by means of the

   _____ .

3. A mechanical device used to restrict a resident's movement is

   called a _____   _____ .

ACTIVITY 3 - IDENTIFY THE RIGHT

For each example, select the resident right which is involved. Write it in on the line below the example.

Right to privacy
Rights to information
Rights to choose
Right to notification of change
Protection of residents' personal
   funds
Grievance rights
Transfer and discharge rights
Right to be free from restraint
   and abuse

1. You notice that a resident is giving out small amounts of cash to other residents.

   _____

2. The resident is uneasy and tries to stay covered up while taking a bath.

   _____

3. The resident is about to be transferred to another wing of the facility.

   _____

4. A resident's daughter wants to see his medical record and care plan.

   _____

5. A staff member loses their temper and grabs a resident's arm.

   _____

6. A resident's family wants to put their complaints in writing.

   _____

7. A resident doesn't like the way a medication makes them feel; they refuse to take it.

   _____

8. A resident wants to maintain contact with friends from her church.

   _____

ACTIVITY 4 – MULTIPLE CHOICE

Circle the letter by the best answer.

1. Residents of nursing facilities have the same rights as:
   A. All children.
   B. All U.S. citizens.
   C. All human beings.
   D. All doctors.

2. Mrs. Ludlow asks to see her financial records and have them explained to her. She is exercising her right to:
   A. Privacy.
   B. Information.
   C. Confidentiality.
   D. Self-determination.

3. A resident must be told that they are to be discharged or transferred:
   A. As soon as staff is told.
   B. One day before the move.
   C. At least 30 days in advance.
   D. At least 2 hours in advance.

4. Screening of potential nurse assistants may include:
   A. Inspection of their wardrobe.
   B. Checks of family members.
   C. Home safety inspection.
   D. Criminal background checks.

5. Mr. Chang returns to his room and discovers he has a new roommate. Which of his rights has been violated?
   A. Right to information.
   B. Right to exercise one's rights.
   C. Right to notification of change.
   D. Right to privacy and confidentiality.

ACTIVITY 5 – MATCHING

Read the examples of abuse. Place the letter of the correct term for that form of abuse next to the example.

Term

A. Theft
B. Neglect
C. Physical abuse
D. Corporal punishment
E. Involuntary seclusion
F. Mental abuse
G. Negligence
H. Verbal abuse
I. Chemical restraint
J. Sexual abuse
K. Physical restraint

Example

1. _____ A resident is shaken by an angry nurse assistant.

2. _____ A bed-ridden resident is not turned as often as they should be.

3. _____ A resident is sedated so they won't wander.

4. _____ Making fun of a resident.

5. _____ Punishing a resident by slapping them.

6. _____ Locking a resident in a room against their will.

7. _____ Allowing one resident to touch another in a sexual way.

8. _____ Stealing a resident's money.

9. _____ Using a device that forces a resident to remain seated.

10. _____ Making a threatening remark to a resident.

11. _____ Failing to do what another nurse assistant would do in the same situation.

ACTIVITY 6 – FILL IN THE BLANK

Belittles
Coercion
Discrimination
Grievance
Interference
Ombudsman
Retaliation

Using the word list above, complete each sentence with the correct term.

1. A resident's family wants to file a formal complaint, called a(n) _____ , because of an accident involving their

    family member.

2. Mrs. Shea has confided to you about an act of _____ she suffered on another shift. The staff member forced her to

    take a bath when she didn't want to, by threatening to tear up one of Mrs. Shea's family photos.

3. Mr. Logan complained to the nurse about a dietary employee who stole money from his wallet. In an act of _____ .

    the employee serves his food cold.

4. If you try to prevent a resident or family member from making a complaint, you would be guilty of _____ .

5. Mrs. McDougal has been excited about attending a special holiday event in the activity room. But because she is blind, the staff doesn't take
    her to the event. The staff is guilty of _____ .

6. When Mrs. Duffy says unkind or hurtful remarks to her roommate, she _____ her.

7. A(n) _____ is required by law to investigate complaints or violations of a resident's rights.

ACTIVITY 7 – QUESTIONS TO CONSIDER

1. Imagine you are a resident in a long term care facility. Which right(s) would you be willing to give up?

2. Describe the difference between a residents' needs and residents' rights.

Chapter 5

NURSE ASSISTANT'S ROLE IN QUALITY OF LIFE

ACTIVITY 1 – WORD SCRAMBLE

Based on the example provided, unscramble each key term and spell it correctly in the spaces directly below.

Alternative   Dignity   Habitat   Perception   Single-minded

1. Even thought you don't know him very well, you always think of your neighbor as being happy and content. This is your <u>mental image</u> of him.

    R O C P E P T E N I   _ _ _ _ _ _ . _ _ _ _

2. Instead of going to work the same way as usual, you choose a new route, <u>a different possibility</u>.

    A N E T I R V A L T E   _ _ _ _ _ _ _ _ _ _ _

3. Until you saw your boss at the mall with her family last Saturday, you never thought about her having a life outside of work. <u>You only saw her in one way.</u>

    E G L S N I – M E D N I D   _ _ _ _ _ _ – _ _ _ _ _ _

4. When you care for Mrs. Fielding based on your knowledge of her needs and preferences and personal history, you <u>convey a feeling of self-worth to her.</u>

    T I G I D Y N   _ _ _ _ _ _ _

5. An Eden alternative facility seeks to create an environment where <u>plants and animals are a natural part of the environment.</u>

    T H I B T A A   _ _ _ _ _ _ _

ACTIVITY 2 – TRUE/FALSE

In the space provided, write in T for true or F for false.

1. _____ As a nurse assistant, you influence a resident's feelings of happiness and wellbeing.

2. _____ New residents will understand if you don't have time to get to know them right away.

3. _____ Thinking of Mr. Roberts as always being cranky and combative can affect how well you care for him.

4. _____ Once you've talked to the charge nurse and reviewed the care plan, you know all you need to know about a new resident in your care.

5. _____ Mrs. Seaver is sad about being in a nursing facility. You can help her by being supportive and allowing her to talk about her feelings.

6. _____ We are all products of our culture, environment, and life experiences.

7. _____ The best way to treat a resident is the way they want to be treated.

8. _____ Staff's perceptions of residents are almost always accurate.

9. _____ The Eden alternative is a theme park based on stories from the Bible.

10. _____ Giving a resident a nickname without their permission is a sign of disrespect.

ACTIVITY 3 – MULTIPLE CHOICE

Circle the letter beside the best answer.

1. Your perception of a resident can be affected by:
   A. Their favorite color.
   B. A hot and humid day.
   C. Your own values and culture.
   D. The resident's clothing choices.

2. What is the BEST way to support a resident's quality of life?
   A. Style their hair in a new way.
   B. Knock on their door as you open it.
   C. Treat them with dignity and respect.
   D. Be friendly whenever their family visits.

3. The goal of activities is to:
   A. Keep the activities director employed.
   B. Help residents become actively engaged.
   C. Make decorations for all national holidays.
   D. Give nurse assistants a few minutes of free time.

4. The goal of an Eden alternative nursing facility is to:
   A. Plant flower and vegetable gardens.
   B. Allow residents to care for plants and pets.
   C. Eliminate loneliness, helplessness, and boredom.
   D. Operate daycare centers and after-school programs.

5. What is the most important part of a nurse assistant's job?
   A. Getting everything done.
   B. Meeting all the resident's needs.
   C. Helping the resident get dressed.
   D. Seeing that residents get fed on time.

ACTIVITY 4 – YES OR NO

Beside each example, write YES if the resident's dignity is promoted, or NO if the resident's dignity is not promoted.

1. _____ Ask permission before giving care to the resident.

2. _____ Call the resident by their preferred name.

3. _____ Insist that the resident wear an outfit you've chosen.

4. _____ Be considerate of the resident's needs, wants, and rights.

5. _____ Rush the resident through their morning care.

6. _____ Take the resident to an activity they won't understand.

7. _____ Treat the resident like a customer.

8. _____ Respect the resident's values, culture, and religion.

9. _____ Leave the door open while the resident gets dressed.

10. _____ Take an interest in the resident's stories.

11. _____ Use baby talk when speaking to the resident.

12. _____ Offer the resident choices.

13. _____ Ask for permission to enter the resident's room.

14. _____ Answer the resident's call light promptly.

15. _____ Touch the resident's belongings without permission.

ACTIVITY 5 – MATCHING

Match the situation with the appropriate reaction. Write the letter for the response in the space by the situation.

Situation

1. _____ You enter Mr. Galanos' room and, as usual, he has something to complain about.

2. _____ Mrs. Hanak doesn't attend any activities and seems depressed.

3. _____ You have tried before to address Mrs. Lemley's concerns about her meals, even though you don't work in dietary. Today she isn't happy with her lunch.

4. _____ Mrs. Adkins is using a walker today, after having been wheelchair bound for over a week.

5. _____ Your new resident has been very quiet. You learn from his roommate that he is a football fan.

Response

A. As you care for him, start a conversation about football. Encourage him to share his opinions about the sport.

B. Praise the resident for their progress.

C. Remember that the resident has chronic back pain and recently lost his son.

D. Using a pleasant tone of voice, ask the resident what they would like changed about their meal, and work with dietary staff to satisfy their needs.

E. Encourage them to talk. Ask about his/her past, family, hobbies, and talents.

1. Why is dignity important to residents?

2. Describe a situation in which you were not treated with dignity. How did you feel?

3. What do you think happens to residents when they are not treated with dignity?

4. If a resident is unhappy with some aspect of their care, what can they expect from you?

Chapter 6

THE ROLE OF THE FAMILY

Read each question. Choose the key term that answers the question and write that term on the line provided.

Family   Feedback   Guilt   Stress

1. When someone has committed an offense or believes they have done something wrong to another person, what emotion might they feel?

    _____

2. What is the term for people who are important to a resident, or related to the resident by marriage or ancestry?

    _____

3. When someone has a physical or emotional reaction to an event or situation, and that reaction causes them mental tension, what is the reaction called?

    _____

4. When we receive information that is corrective or evaluative, what is that information called?

    _____

ACTIVITY 2 - MULTIPLE CHOICE

Circle the letter beside the best answer.

1. The family will be happy with the care you provide their relative if they know:
   A. You provide care quickly.
   B. You follow most of the facility's policies.
   C. You provide good care with compassion.
   D. You always greet them with a friendly smile.

2. A family can be an important resource for you because:
   A. They can shop for the resident.
   B. They can bring special foods for the resident.
   C. They know the resident better than anyone else.
   D. They keep the resident occupied when they visit.

3. Each new resident and family goes through an adjustment process that lasts until:
   A. The resident stops complaining.
   B. The family has come to terms with its guilt.
   C. The resident is participating in all activities in the facility.
   D. Everyone is comfortable and a trusting relationship has developed.

4. You will get along with a resident's family if you see them as:
   A. Someone you can socialize with outside of work.
   B. Having total control over the happiness of their loved one.
   C. Someone who should give all the personal care to the resident.
   D. A partner with whom you share common goals and decision making.

5. If a family member criticizes the care their resident has received, you should:
   A. Explain to the family that they are wrong to be concerned.
   B. Tell them to move the resident immediately to another facility.
   C. Listen carefully to their concerns and correct any problems you can.
   D. Assume that they still feel guilty about moving their relative into the facility.

ACTIVITY 3 - TRUE/FALSE

Write T for True or F for False in the blank next to each example.

1. _____ A new resident in a nursing facility goes through an adjustment process.

2. _____ The new resident's family always feels a sense of relief.

3. _____ You should be careful not to judge what a family says or does.

4. _____ The term significant others means anyone who is important to the resident.

5. _____ The resident is your only customer, not the family.

6. _____ Family members are important mostly because they bring in the resident's favorite foods.

7. _____ Families should not be allowed to help with their family member's care.

8. _____ Some residents have difficult or stressful relationships with family members.

9. _____ Families rarely feel sad when their loved one moves into a nursing facility.

10. _____ Feedback from families is always negative.

ACTIVITY 4 – CASE STUDY

Read the following situations and circle the best response in the following questions.

1. Mrs. Chesnutt, a resident in your care, has emphysema and her health is failing. Her daughter has been critical of her mother's care during her last two visits. She believes staff could be doing more to help her mother improve. What should you say to her?
    A. "I give your mother the best care I can."
    B. "You need to accept the fact that your mother isn't going to get better."
    C. "I can see that you're worried, and I'm sorry you have concerns. Would you like for me to get the charge nurse?"

2. Mr. Lomax is a new resident. He is angry that his family has put him in a nursing facility. When his family members come to visit, he barely speaks to them. What can you say to make the family feel better?
    A. "Mr. Lomax will adjust before you know it."
    B. "This is just a phase. Why don't you put off your next visit until he's had time to adjust?"
    C. "Mr. Lomax is getting the very best care. Is there anything we can do to make your visits more pleasant?"

3. Mrs. White's daughter likes to bring her mother home-cooked foods. But recently the doctor prescribed a low-salt diet, which would mean an end to her meals of collard greens and green beans with bacon. If Mrs. White and her daughter refuse to cooperate, what should you do?
    A. Don't say anything.
    B. Report the situation to the charge nurse.
    C. Remind them about the doctor's orders, but don't insist on their cooperation.

4. Mrs. Cadden's daughter wants to help transfer her mother from the bed to a wheelchair. She insists that the way they did it at home is safer for her mother than the method staff uses. What should you say?
    A. "There is no way I can allow you to do that."
    B. "Let me get the charge nurse so she can review the transfer."
    C. "Go ahead and move her, but the facility isn't responsible if she falls."

5. Mrs. Hearn has just returned to the facility from the hospital. She is weak and must be in a wheelchair because of her brief illness. The doctor's orders are for staff to begin ambulating her 3 times a day using a walker. Her son is visiting and tells you it is too soon for his mother to be walking. What should you say?
    A. "I'm sorry, Mr. Hearn, but I've got orders to walk your mother. It's my job and I'm going to do it."
    B. "I know you're concerned, but your mother will continue to lose strength if she doesn't start walking."
    C. "I know I'm right about this, Mr. Hearn. I think you should step out of the room."

ACTIVITY 5 – IN YOUR OWN WORDS

1. Think about the most important people in your life. Also think about what it would it mean to them and to you if you had to put them in a long term care facility. How do you think they would feel?

How would you feel?

What would you do to make them feel better?

2. List 3 things you can do to help family members adjust to the facility and the care their loved one is receiving.

3. How do you respond to families who:

Are uncomfortable visiting

Seem bossy

Are upset

Are arguing with each other

Chapter 7

COMMUNICATION

ACTIVITY 1 – FILL IN THE BLANK

Complete each sentence with the correct medical or key term.

Aphasia
Avoidance
Clarify
Cognitive impairment
Collaboration

Communication
Competition
Compromise
Condolences
Conflict resolution

Context
Curtness
Diversion
Nickname
Nonverbal communication

Smirking
Surname
Tact
Validated

1. An agreement in which both parties agree to give up something is called a(n) _____ .

2. Something is _____ when it is proven to be valid, sound, or effective.

3. _____ is the art of saying the appropriate and polite thing at the right time.

4. _____ is a brusque, impolite manner of speaking to someone.

5. When someone has difficulty putting thoughts into words, they have a condition called _____ .

6. A person's last name is also known as their _____ .

7. Expressions of sorrow or sympathy are known as _____ .

8. Anything that distracts a person's attention is called a(n) _____ .

9. _____ is the term for sending and receiving messages verbally and nonverbally.

10. Understanding the whole situation, background, or _____ helps to give meaning to someone's words.

11. People are in _____ when they try to beat each other to a goal.

12. The act of working together is called _____.

13. Resolving problems through the use of effective communication is called _____.

14. Escaping from an issue, rather than dealing with it, is called _____.

15. Sending a message without the use of words is done by _____.

16. Family and friends often call each other by special names, called _____.

17. The term for smiling at someone in a way that suggests you feel superior to that person is _____.

18. We _____ something, in order to make sure it is clearly understood.

19. When a person's ability to think, remember, or solve problems has been changed or damaged, they have a(n) _____.

ACTIVITY 2 – DO'S & DON'TS

In the space beside each example, write "Do" if it is an example of good communication and "Don't" if it is a bad example.

1. _____ Use a pleasant tone when you speak.

2. _____ Make eye contact when you speak and when you listen.

3. _____ Talk with food or gum in your mouth.

4. _____ Speak clearly and slowly.

5. _____ Use terms that the resident will understand.

6. _____ Reduce or eliminate other sounds such as radio or TV.

7. _____ Roll your eyes.

8. _____ Stop what you are doing to listen.

9. _____ Turn your back on the person you're talking with.

10. _____ Use medical terms or slang words.

11. _____ Give residents nicknames.

12. _____ Cover your mouth with your hand as you speak.

13. _____ Validate what the person is saying by nodding or agreeing.

14. _____ Clarify what's been said by repeating it in your own words.

15. _____ Fold your arms across your chest.

ACTIVITY 3 – MULTIPLE CHOICE

Circle the letter beside the best answer.

1. A confused resident is behaving aggressively toward his roommate. As a nurse assistant, you should:
   A. Run down the hall to get the charge nurse.
   B. In a firm tone of voice, tell the resident to be quiet.
   C. Smile and talk in a friendly voice as you approach the resident.
   D. Approach the resident quickly and pull them into another room.

2. You are involved in a disagreement with a co-worker. In order to resolve the conflict, you should:
   A. Change the subject.
   B. Bluntly say what you feel.
   C. Avoid reacting defensively.
   D. Tell the co-worker they are wrong.

3. A new resident's family is very demanding, and you cannot seem to satisfy them. You should:
   A. Try to ignore their requests.
   B. Refer them to the charge nurse.
   C. Ask the resident to talk with them.
   D. Remember that work will be over soon.

4. If you want to be an effective listener for a resident in your care, you should NOT:
   A. Nod as they talk.
   B. Validate what they are saying.
   C. Maintain eye contact with them.
   D. Encourage them to tell their story quickly.

5. If a resident or family member asks you to talk about yourself, you should:
   A. Share your complete family medical history.
   B. Ask them for advice about a personal problem.
   C. Tell a brief story similar to one the resident told you.
   D. Describe a difficult financial situation you are facing.

ACTIVITY 4 – SITUATION/STATEMENT

Read each situation. In the space provided, write the letter of the appropriate statement.

Situation

1. _____ Mrs. Hooper wants to show you new photos of her great-granddaughter, but you have 4 more residents to assist with personal care.

2. _____ A nurse assistant has confided to you about a serious personal problem. You don't feel qualified to give her advice.

3. _____ A family member has arrived before her mother has had morning care. She criticizes you about her mother's appearance.

4. _____ Mr. Pierce has kept to himself since he was admitted 2 weeks ago. You notice that he participated in a current events activity this morning.

5. _____ Mrs. McDonald usually enjoys getting exercise. Today she cringed when you suggested taking a walk to the end of the hallway.

Statement

A. "Are you not feeling well today? It's important for you to tell me if something is wrong."

B. "It's great to see you out of your room. I hope you'll participate in more activities."

C. "She certainly is a beautiful child. I'd like to see all your photos, but I still have residents to care for. What if I come back later when I have more time to spend with you?"

D. "I give each resident all the time and assistance they need to look and feel their best each day. I'm sorry your mother hasn't had her morning care yet, but I have time now to help her bathe and dress."

E. "I know you must be in a lot of pain over your situation. Have you thought about talking to your pastor or a counselor?"

1. What are 5 ways to promote effective communication?

_____

_____

_____

_____

_____

2. What are 2 specific techniques that can improve communication with residents who have these impairments?

   A. Visual impairment

_____

_____

_____

   B. Hearing loss

_____

_____

_____

C. Depression or withdrawal

_____

_____

_____

D. Speech impairment

_____

_____

_____

E. Memory loss

_____

_____

_____

3. Describe a situation when someone's non-verbal message didn't match their verbal message.

_____

_____

_____

_____

Chapter 8

DOCUMENTATION PRINCIPLES AND PROCEDURES

ACTIVITY 1 – FILL IN THE BLANK

Complete each sentence with the correct term.

Assessment
Care plan
Documentation

Minimum data set (MDS)
Objective
Quality indicators

Resident Assessment Instrument (RAI)
Resident assessment protocols (RAPS)
Subjective

1. The _____ _____ _____ contains resident information on the RAI, including levels of physical functioning and bladder and bowel continence.

2. Information is _____ when it is based on a hunch you may have about a resident, or it is something the resident tells you they are feeling.

3. A summary of an entire facility's MDS information is called _____, and indicates the quality of care provided at the facility.

4. Any written reports maintained by a facility are called _____.

5. A written interdisciplinary document, called the _____, lists the resident's needs and goals, along with the actions and approaches the staff will take to help the resident meet those goals.

6. The _____ _____ is a tool used by long term care facilities to document key information about residents including their care plans and outcomes.

7. An evaluation of a patient or condition is called an _____.

8. Information that is based on fact, and that everyone will agree with is called _____.

9. The _____ _____ _____ section of the RAI includes a more detailed assessment of problem areas.

Match the item or type of information with the report or record where that information is contained. Some reports or records may be used more than once.

Type of Information	Report or Record
Type of Information	**Report or Record**
1. _____ Needs, goals, and approaches for improving a resident's condition.	A. Care plan
2. _____ A description of an accident involving a resident.	B. Flow sheet
3. _____ Admission papers.	C. RAPS
4. _____ Daily records of a resident's intake and output (I & O).	D. Quality indicators
5. _____ A section of the RAI that has a more detailed assessment of a resident's problems.	E. MDS
6. _____ A summary of statistics about residents and the quality of care they receive at a facility.	F. Medical record
7. _____ Results of a resident's lab tests.	G. Incident report
8. _____ Written guidelines for handling a resident's personal belongings.	H. RAI
9. _____ An assessment of a resident's levels of functioning which is completed by staff in several departments.	I. Policies and procedures
10. _____ Five components including MDS, RAPS, care plan development, care plan implementation, and evaluation & outcome.	
11. _____ A nurse assistant scraped her arm as she reached for a slipper under a resident's bed.	

ACTIVITY 3 — TRUE/FALSE

In the space provided, write T for true or F for false.

1. _____ A resident's medical record belongs to their family.

2. _____ The care plan is another name for the medical record.

3. _____ Physical and occupational therapists may add information to a resident's chart.

4. _____ Some facilities use words and symbols on resident's door cards to communicate important information.

5. _____ Hunches are based on factual information.

6. _____ "This resident is 5'4" tall" is a subjective statement.

7. _____ Good observations should include detailed objective and subjective information.

8. _____ A nurse assistant plays a vital role in the assessment of a resident's condition.

9. _____ The least important assessment tool a facility uses is the Resident Assessment Instrument (RAI).

10. _____ The RAI must be completed for all Medicare/Medicaid residents.

11. _____ "Quality indicators" sum up the quality of care a facility provides all its residents.

12. _____ Resident care plans are revised every 6 months.

13. _____ Routine reporting is usually done just before the charge nurse goes to lunch.

14. _____ It is important for you to watch for changes in your residents' health.

15. _____ You should know your facility's policies on documentation before you write in a resident's chart.

ACTIVITY 4 — MULTIPLE CHOICE

Circle the letter by the best answer.

1. The MDS and RAPS are parts of the:
   A. RAI.
   B. Care plan.
   C. Incident report.
   D. Quality indicators.

2. You should check with the charge nurse before you share medical information about a resident with:
   A. The dietitian.
   B. The resident's family.
   C. The physical therapist.
   D. The resident's physician.

3. Which of the following items will a typical resident care plan include?
   A. Graphs or flow sheets of vital signs.
   B. Needs, goals, and approaches to care.
   C. Permission forms signed by the resident.
   D. Progress notes from the occupational therapist.

4. As you talk to a resident about their care, you should always use:
   A. Hand gestures.
   B. Correct medical terminology.
   C. Abbreviations of medical terms.
   D. Simple terms the resident will understand.

5. What is the proper way to correct a documentation error?
   A. Erase the entry.
   B. Use "white out" on the entry.
   C. Cross through the entry with a single line.
   D. Cross through the entry with a heavy black marker.

Match each situation with the appropriate response.

Situation	Response
1. _____ Your co-worker has to leave early and asks you to document her residents' conditions.	A. Ask the resident for more details about what happened. Report all this information to the charge nurse so that the right actions can be taken.
2. _____ A resident has made plans to go out to dinner with her family. You're not sure if any forms should be filled out.	B. Make a large "X" over the entire progress note and write "wrong resident" in the margin with your initials.
3. _____ A resident's roommate reports that the resident slipped off the toilet. The resident says "I didn't fall all the way to the floor and I'm okay!" You don't see any bruising or injuries.	C. Repeat your statement using simple terms, "Your doctor wants you to go to physical therapy twice today."
4. _____ You have just written a lengthy progress note in a resident's chart when you realize it's the wrong chart.	D. You are only allowed to document your own actions and observations. Remind your co-worker that it is illegal for you to document for anyone else.
5. _____ You have just told a resident they have orders to go to physical therapy BID. They stare at you and appear confused.	E. You share your thoughts, ideas, and suggestions in a tactful and respectful manner.
6. _____ You are asked to participate in a resident's care planning meeting.	F. Every facility should have a policy and procedure document about residents leaving the facility. Obtain a copy of the policy and follow each step correctly.

ACTIVITY 6 — IMMEDIATE REPORTING/ROUTINE REPORTING

Read the following list of observations. In the space provided, write an I if you would report the observation immediately. If you would report the observation during routine reporting, write an R.

1. _____ You find a resident lying on the floor. They appear to have fallen.

2. _____ Mrs. Lindsey has a fresh and bleeding skin tear on her arm.

3. _____ A resident's urine is dark and cloudy.

4. _____ Mrs. McKenzie says, "I feel a little down today."

5. _____ A resident has not had a bowel movement for 2 days.

6. _____ A resident tells you she sees snakes on her bed. There are no snakes on her bed, and she has never said anything like this before.

Chapter

PREVENTION AND CONTROL OF INFECTION

Write the letter of the definition next to the key term it defines.

Term	Definition
1. _____ Airborne transmission	A. a condition of being in direct or indirect contact with an infectious microorganism
2. _____ Barrier	B. openings in the body where microorganisms can enter
3. _____ Direct transmission	C. transmission of infection by an intermediate object, such as food, water, medical equipment, or a person's hands, to the portal of entry of a susceptible host
4. _____ Exposure	D. something that impedes or separates a person from an infectious microorganism
5. _____ Indirect transmission	E. direct transfer of microorganisms from one person to another
6. _____ Portal of entry	F. a person, animal, or environment in which an infectious agent lives
7. _____ Reservoir	G. transfer an infectious agent from one person or place to another
8. _____ Transmit	H. route of transmission occurs when the reservoir coughs microorganisms into the air and a susceptible host breathes them into the lungs

ACTIVITY 2 – SPELL IT OUT

Using the word list below and the definition provided in each example, complete the spelling of the term.

Antibiotics   Hepatitis   Microorganism   Syphilis
Bacteria   Human immunodeficiency virus   Nonpathogenic   Tuberculosis
Fungi   Immunization   Pathogenic   Virus
Gonorrhea   Infection   Standard precautions

1. Infection of the liver.

   H __ P __ __ __ __ __ __

2. A kind of microorganism like yeast and mold.

   __ __ __ G I

3. Microorganisms or substances that can produce disease.

   __ __ T H __ G __ __ __ C

4. Recommendations from CDC for facilities to use in handling blood, body fluids, secretion, excretion (except sweat), nonintact skin such as cuts and wounds, and mucous membranes of all residents, to prevent infection.

   S __ __ __ D __ __ D

   P __ __ C __ __ T __ __ N __

5. Infectious, bacterial, communicable disease primarily affecting the lungs, also known as TB.

   T __ B __ __ C __ L __ __ __ __

6. Contagious bacterial venereal infection that is sexually transmitted.

   G __ N __ __ R H __ __

7. Condition produced when an infective agent becomes established in or on a suitable host.

   __ N F __ __ __ __ __ N

8. Drugs that reduce or kill microorganisms.

   __ N __ B __ T __ __ __ __

9. One-celled microorganisms that may cause infection.

   B __ __ T __ R __ __

10. Microorganisms that do not cause infection.

    N __ __ P __ __ __ __ G __ __ __ C

11. Viral infection transmitted by contact with blood and other body fluids such as semen and vaginal secretions, also known as HIV.

    __ __ __ M __ N

    I __ M __ __ __ D __ __ __ __ __ __ N __ __

    V __ R __ __

12. A type of microorganism that survives only in living things.

    __ __ R __ S

13. Virus, bacteria, or fungus that cannot be seen with the naked eye; also called a germ.

    __ __ C __ __ __ R G __ __ __ __ M

14. A chronic contagious venereal infection that is sexually transmitted.

    __ Y __ __ __ L __ __

15. Administration of a vaccine to make the person immune (not susceptible) to a specific infection.

    __ __ M __ __ Z __ T __ __ __

ACTIVITY 3 – FILL IN THE BLANK

Using the terms provided, complete each sentence correctly.

Biohazard   Contaminated   Invasive   Sanitation
Condom   Disinfectant   Isolation   Sterilization

1. An agent that inactivates microorganisms on inanimate objects is called a(n) _____ .

2. If something is impure or unclean, it is _____ .

3. _____ is the term for something that enters the body.

4. _____ is the promotion of hygiene and prevention of disease by maintaining clean conditions.

5. A(n) _____ is a thin, flexible sheath commonly made of latex rubber, worn over the penis to reduce the risk of pregnancy and transmission of sexually transmitted diseases

6. When someone is set apart from others, they are in _____ .

7. _____ causes the complete elimination or destruction of all microbial life.

8. A(n) _____ is anything that is harmful or potentially harmful to humans or the environment.

ACTIVITY 4 – CHAIN OF INFECTION

In the diagram below, write the six steps/conditions in the chain of infection in the order by which infection occurs.

Microorganism   Portal of exit   Susceptible host
Portal of entry   Reservoir   Transmission

6th _____   1st _____

5th _____   2nd _____

4th _____   3rd _____

ACTIVITY 5 – DIRECT/INDIRECT

Review each action. If transmission of infection could be made directly by the action, write D in the space provided. Write I if the transmission would be indirect.

1. _____ Coughing

2. _____ Sneezing

3. _____ Shaking hands

4. _____ Changing dressings

5. _____ Carrying dirty linen

6. _____ Opening doors

7. _____ Eating contaminated food

8. _____ Kissing

9. _____ Sexual intercourse

10. _____ Picking up soiled tissues

ACTIVITY 6 – TRUE/FALSE

Write a T for True or an F for False by each statement.

1. _____ The most important way to prevent the spread of infection is by washing your hands.

2. _____ It is important to rinse your hands from your fingertips down to your wrists after you've washed them with soap.

3. _____ Use standard precautions whenever you might come in contact with a resident's bodily fluids.

4. _____ The OSHA Bloodborne Pathogen Standard is intended to protect workers from HIV, hepatitis B, and hepatitis C.

5. _____ Single-use gloves can be reused if they don't look dirty.

6. _____ A disinfectant should be used to clean up blood or other bodily fluids.

7. _____ You don't need to wash your hands after a procedure if you were wearing gloves.

8. _____ If a resident is on isolation precautions, only a nurse can provide their care.

9. _____ All objects that have been used by a resident or caregiver are considered dirty.

10. _____ Residents who are on isolation precautions may need emotional support from staff and family.

ACTIVITY 7 – MULTIPLE CHOICE

Circle the best answer to each statement or question.

1. Bacteria is a type of:
   A. Fungi.
   B. Influenza.
   C. Antibiotic.
   D. Microorganism.

2. A microorganism that cannot cause infection is:
   A. Bacteria.
   B. Antibiotic.
   C. Pathogenic.
   D. Nonpathogenic.

3. Mrs. Reynolds had surgery recently and is at risk of getting an infection. In the chain of infection, what is she called?
   A. Reservoir.
   B. Portal of exit.
   C. Portal of entry.
   D. Susceptible host.

4. The goal of standard precautions is to:
   A. Prevent residents and staff from slipping or falling down.
   B. Prevent residents from wandering away from the facility.
   C. Prevent the airborne transmission of the cold and flu viruses.
   D. Prevent the transmission of diseases when handling bodily fluids.

5. Direct transmission of a microorganism occurs by:
   A. Handling soiled linens.
   B. Using a contaminated phone.
   C. Kissing or sexual intercourse.
   D. Eating off someone else's plate.

INJURY PREVENTION

Chapter 10

ACTIVITY 1 – MATCHING

In the space provided, write the letter of the correct definition.

Term	Definition
1. _____ Biceps	A. Moving residents out of the facility to another site for safety.
2. _____ Body mechanics	B. Written information sheets describing chemicals used in a facility.
3. _____ Ergonomics	C. Strong arm muscles used for lifting.
4. _____ External evacuation	D. Moving residents to another section within the facility for safety.
5. _____ Internal evacuation	E. Principles of using your body efficiently to do something.
6. _____ Material safety data sheets (MSDS)	F. Study of relationships between workers' physical capabilities and their job tasks.

ACTIVITY 2 – SAFE & UNSAFE

Read each example. In the blank provided, write an S if the example is a safe practice or a U if it is an unsafe practice.

1. _____ Wait for housekeeping to clean up a small spill in the hallway.

2. _____ Consider your own strength and body mechanics before you move a resident.

3. _____ Respond to a resident's call light when you have the time.

4. _____ Wear nonskid shoes.

5. _____ Turn the hallway lights off at night.

6. _____ Leave the resident's slippers by their bed in case they get up in the night.

7. _____ Consider the resident's capabilities before you transfer them.

8. _____ Bend your knees and lift using your leg and arm muscles, not your back.

9. _____ Get a good grip on the resident by holding on to their shirt collar.

10. _____ Remove unnecessary items from the resident's room and bathroom.

11. _____ Set up a new resident's radio using an extension cord.

12. _____ If a resident gets a chemical on their skin, rinse it off with lots of running water.

13. _____ Lean an empty oxygen tank against the wall, outside a resident's room

14. _____ Handle bottles of hazardous chemicals when you don't know their contents.

ACTIVITY 3 – MULTIPLE CHOICE.

Circle the letter beside the best answer.

1. What is the FIRST step in the 5-step approach to preventing injuries when caring for a resident?
   A. Follow the care plan.
   B. Determine the resident's capabilities.
   C. Determine the equipment you will need.
   D. Evaluate the success of the tasks you have performed.

2. Pivot discs are used to help a resident:
   A. Exercise
   B. Use a walker.
   C. Transfer from the bed to chair.
   D. Perform range-of-motion exercises.

3. If you enter a room where there is a fire, what should you do FIRST?
   A. Stop and quickly assess the situation.
   B. Immediately remove all residents from the area.
   C. When everyone is out, close the door to the room.
   D. Yell for help and sound an alarm if one is present.

4. What is the hug position?
   A. A policy having to do with affection between residents.
   B. Holding an object or person close to you as you move them.
   C. Two nurse assistants hug the resident from either side as they lift.
   D. A means of limiting inappropriate behaviors between staff and residents.

5. A resident's bed should be kept in its lowest position when:
   A. You are changing the sheets.
   B. You are giving the resident a bed bath.
   C. The resident is resting in the bed or the bed is empty.
   D. Family is coming to visit and there aren't enough chairs.

ACTIVITY 4 – SHOULD & SHOULD NOT

Read each example. In the blank provided, write an S if the example is a step you SHOULD take or a SN if it is step you SHOULD NOT take in the event of a fire.

1. _____ Attempt to put out a fire that is climbing up a wall.

2. _____ Attempt to put out a small fire in a trashcan.

3. _____ Open the windows in a room where there's a fire.

4. _____ Use oxygen to put out a fire.

5. _____ Remove residents from a room where there is a fire and close the door.

6. _____ Yell for help, and sound an alarm if present.

7. _____ Open a door when you see smoke coming from underneath it.

8. _____ Evacuate residents at immediate risk to the end of the farthest wing from the fire.

9. _____ Throw water on a large fire.

10. _____ Close the door to a room that's on fire.

ACTIVITY 5 – MATCHING

Match each example of safety documentation to the correct term.

Term

1. _____ Access to Employee Exposure and Medical Records Standard

2. _____ Material safety data sheet (MSDS)

3. _____ Incident report

Example

A. A report on an accident involving staff or residents.

B. A sheet that lists a substance's chemical contents, fire and health hazards, use precautions, clean-up procedures, disposal requirements, needed personal protective equipment, and first aid procedures.

C. An OSHA publication explaining your right to see your medical records, a chemical inventory list, and material safety data sheets.

ACTIVITY 6 – IDEAS TO CONSIDER

1. Make a list of safety rules you were taught as a child, or safety rules you are teaching your children.

2. Of the rules listed above, how many do you practice daily?

3. If you do not practice some of the rules, explain why.

4. Give 2 examples of injuries that can be prevented by following one of your own safety rules.

Chapter 11

THE AGING PROCESS AND DISEASE MANAGEMENT

ACTIVITY 1 – MATCHING

Match the letter next to each definition with the correct term for that definition.

1. _____ Endocrine system

2. _____ Insulin

3. _____ Pituitary gland

4. _____ Sebaceous glands

5. _____ Testes (testicles)

A. body system made up of many glands that secrete hormones

B. glands that are located in the dermis and secrete oil

C. the two oval glands that manufacture sperm cells and the male sex hormone testosterone

D. hormone involved in breaking down carbohydrates in the body

E. a gland located in the brain that secretes hormones and regulates other glands

ACTIVITY 2 – FILL IN THE BLANK

Complete each sentence using the correct term.

Arteries   Circulatory system   Edema
Capillaries   Coronary artery disease   Peripheral vascular disease
Cerebral vascular accident   Congestive heart failure   Veins

1. _____ _____ _____ is a condition that causes a diminished blood flow to the arms and legs.

2. The blood vessels that carry deoxygenated blood from the body back to the heart and lungs are called _____ .

3. _____ are tiny blood vessels that connect arteries and veins, where oxygen is exchanged for carbon dioxide inside organs.

4. The body system that includes the heart and blood vessels that carry oxygen and nutrients to the body and remove carbon dioxide is called the _____ _____ .

5. _____ _____ _____ is a condition that results in reduced blood flow through the coronary arteries, which nourish the heart.

6. Swelling, or _____ , because of fluid gain or retention, is most commonly observed in the legs and ankles.

7. When the blood flow to the brain is interrupted (also called stroke), a(n) _____ _____ _____ occurs.

8. _____ are blood vessels that carry oxygenated blood to all parts of the body.

9. _____ _____ _____ is a condition that occurs when the heart muscle weakens and the heart becomes ineffective in moving blood through the body.

ACTIVITY 3 – FILL IN THE BLANK

Complete each sentence using the correct term.

Digestive system
Constipation
Enema
Fecal impaction

1. _____ is the condition in which bowel movement is delayed and feces are difficult to expel from the rectum.

2. _____ may occur when constipation is not treated; hard feces are impacted in the rectum.

3. The body system that provides the body with a continuous supply of nutrients and fluid and removes waste products is called the

_____ _____ .

4. The procedure known as an _____ introduces fluid into the rectum to stimulate a bowel movement.

ACTIVITY 4 – SPELL IT OUT

Using the terms provided in the box, spell out each word beside the correct description.

Blister
Dermatitis
Dermis
Epidermis
Integumentary
Malignant
Mole
Subcutaneous
Wart

1. A colored spot on the body: __ __ L __

2. Refers to a tumor or condition that tends to spread abnormal cells: __ __ L __ G __ __ __ __

3. The top or first layer of the skin: E__ __ __ __ __ __ __ S

4. An elevated area of epidermis containing watery liquid: S __ E__

5. The second layer of the skin: __ __ __ M __ __ __

6. The body system made up of the skin, nails, and hair: __ __ T __ __ __ __ __ __ __ R __

7. Under the skin: __ __ B __ __ __ __ __ __ __ S

8. A horny bump on the skin caused by a virus: __ A __ __

9. Inflammation of the skin: __ __ R __ __ __ T __ __

ACTIVITY 5 – FILL IN THE BLANK

Complete each sentence using the correct term.

Arthritis
Fracture
Muscle atrophy
Musculoskeletal system
Osteoarthritis
Osteoporosis
Rheumatoid arthritis

1. Inflammation that causes pain and limits movement in affected joints is called _____.

2. _____ is another term for a broken bone.

3. The _____ _____ is made up of bones, muscles, tendons, ligaments, and joints.

4. Joint inflammation caused by "wear and tear" of the joint is called _____.

5. A condition in which bones become weak and brittle due to loss of minerals, especially calcium, is called _____.

6. _____ _____ is an inflammatory joint disease.

7. When muscle wastes away, it is known as _____ _____.

ACTIVITY 6 – MATCHING

Match the letter next to each definition with the correct term for that definition.

1. _____ Multiple sclerosis

2. _____ Nervous system

3. _____ Parkinson's disease

A. a neurological disease that affects motor skills

B. progressive disabling disease that affects nerve fibers

C. body system made up of the brain, spinal cord, and nerves

ACTIVITY 7 – SPELL IT OUT

Using the terms provided in the box, spell out each word beside the correct description.

Fallopian tubes
Ovaries
Penis
Reproductive
Uterus
Vagina
Vulva

1. A muscular canal in the female involved in sexual intercourse, childbirth, and passage of menstrual flow: __ __ G __ __ __

2. Two tubes that carry egg cells from the ovaries to the uterus: __ __ L __ __ P __ __ __ __ __ B __ __

3. Organs in the female's pelvic area that secrete hormones involved in sexual function and becoming pregnant: __ V __ __ __ __ __

4. Body system that provides sexual pleasure and allows for human reproduction: __ __ P __ __ __ __ __ __ __ V __

5. The external structure of the female sex organs: __ __ __ V __

6. A muscular reproductive organ where the fetus develops during pregnancy; it sheds its lining during menstruation: __ __ E __ __ __

7. Male organ of sexual intercourse and urination: __ __ __ I __

ACTIVITY 8 – MATCHING

Match the letter next to each definition with the correct term for that definition.

1. _____ Alveoli

2. _____ Bronchi

3. _____ Chronic obstructive pulmonary disease

4. _____ Cyanosis

5. _____ Pneumonia

6. _____ Respiratory system

7. _____ Ventilation

A. lung infection

B. body system that takes in oxygen (inhale) and expels carbon dioxide (exhale)

C. air sacs in the lungs

D. chronic inflammatory disease of bronchial passages and lungs; three most common types of disease are bronchitis, emphysema, and asthma

E. process of moving air in and out of lungs

F. right and left airway structures to the lungs

G. a bluish or purplish discoloration of the skin caused by deficient oxygenation of the blood

ACTIVITY 9 – MULTIPLE CHOICE

Circle the letter beside the best answer.

1. A resident who wakes up with swelling and pain in their arthritic knees has:
   A. A symptom of an acute infection.
   B. A compromised immune system.
   C. An acute condition in a chronic phase.
   D. A chronic condition in an acute phase.

2. What is a silent infection?
   A. An infection that lasts a long time.
   B. An infection with dramatic symptoms.
   C. An infection that does not respond to treatment.
   D. An infection that can only be detected through lab tests.

3. Which body system is responsible for maintaining fluid balance and eliminating liquid wastes?
   A. The urinary system.
   B. The nervous system.
   C. The integumentary system.
   D. The musculoskeletal system.

4. How does the circulatory system change with aging?
   A. Brain cells die.
   B. Muscle strength decreases.
   C. Blood vessels become more rigid and stiff.
   D. Chest wall and lung structures become more rigid.

5. The signs and symptoms of cataracts include:
   A. Hearing loss.
   B. Problems with glare.
   C. Blindness in both eyes.
   D. Heightened color sensitivity.

ACTIVITY 10 – LABELING

Label each of the following pictures, based on the body system it represents.

Circulatory System
Digestive System
Endocrine System (Female)

Endocrine System (Male)
Integumentary System
Musculoskeletal System

Nervous System
Reproductive System (Female)
Reproductive System (Male)

Respiratory System
Sensory System
Urinary System

1. _____

2. _____

3. _____

4. _____

5. _____

6. _____

7. _____

8. _____

9. _____

10. _____

11. _____

12. _____

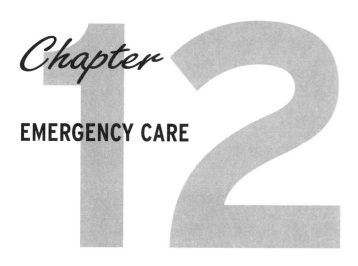

Chapter 12

EMERGENCY CARE

ACTIVITY 1 – MATCHING

In the space provided, write the letter of the description that defines the term.

Term	Definition
1. _____ Aura	A. Excessive loss of blood in a short period of time.
2. _____ Cardiopulmonary resuscitation (CPR)	B. Fatty deposits on blood vessel walls.
3. _____ Cholesterol	C. Breastbone.
4. _____ Heimlich maneuver	D. A substance present in animal cells and body fluids.
5. _____ Hemorrhage	E. Procedure done to dislodge an object from the throat of a choking resident.
6. _____ Palpitations	F. A subtle sensation that often precedes a seizure.
7. _____ Plaque	G. Strong, rapid heartbeats.
8. _____ Protein	H. Procedure to maintain breathing and circulation in a person experiencing cardiac arrest.
9. _____ Seizure	I. Combination of amino acids essential for all living cells.
10. _____ Shock	J. A condition resulting from an abnormality in the brain.
11. _____ Sternum	K. A condition in which vital organs in the body are not getting enough blood and oxygen to maintain good function.

ACTIVITY 2 – TRUE/FALSE

In the space provided, write T for true statements or F for false statements.

1. _____ CPR should be performed on any unconscious resident.

2. _____ Chest pain is a symptom of a seizure.

3. _____ A person is hemorrhaging if they have lost 3 quarts of blood.

4. _____ Unusual thirst can be a symptom of shock.

5. _____ The Heimlich maneuver is done to assist a person in cardiac arrest.

6. _____ When one person does CPR, they should give 2 breaths for every 15 compressions.

7. _____ Residents and visitors always know not to smoke in a room where oxygen is in use.

8. _____ Heart attacks are caused by palpitations.

9. _____ You should not try to hold down a resident having a seizure.

10. _____ It is natural to feel nervous and scared during an emergency.

11. _____ Cardiac arrest can result from a heart attack.

12. _____ An airway obstruction causes a person to stop breathing.

13. _____ Before having a seizure, a resident may feel an aura.

14. _____ Electrical burns are caused by direct exposure to fire.

15. _____ It's important to manage your own feelings in an emergency.

ACTIVITY 3 – LABELING

Using the word list, label the parts of the heart.

Word List

Right atrium
Valve (2)
Left atrium
Aorta
Left ventricle
Right ventricle

1. _____

2. _____

3. _____

4. _____

5. _____

6. _____

7. _____

ACTIVITY 4 – MULTIPLE CHOICE

Circle the letter next to the best answer.

1. In any emergency, a nurse assistant should stay with the resident, call for help, and:
   A. Remain calm.
   B. Always give first aid.
   C. Always give CPR.
   D. Take the resident's pulse.

2. You discover that a resident has a deep cut on their arm. What is the FIRST step you take?
   A. Elevate the arm.
   B. Call for the nurse.
   C. Have the resident lie down.
   D. Clean up any spilled blood.

3. Heart attacks are caused by:
   A. Difficulty breathing.
   B. Weakness and fatigue.
   C. A rapid, weak, irregular pulse.
   D. A blockage in the coronary arteries.

4. Cardiopulmonary resuscitation (CPR) is performed on a resident who:
   A. Is choking.
   B. Has cardiac arrest.
   C. Has cold and clammy skin.
   D. Does not respond to your touch.

5. The ABCs of cardiopulmonary resuscitation include:
   A. Lying the resident on their side.
   B. Giving artificial breathing.
   C. Elevating the lower extremities.
   D. Putting compression on a bleeding wound.

ACTIVITY 5 – LABELING

Using the descriptions provided, label each photo with the letter next to the correct description.

Photo Descriptions

A. Resident choking on food.
B. Nurse assistant giving the Heimlich maneuver to a resident.
C. Nurse assistant holding resident's hand under cool running water.
D. Nurse assistant opening a resident's airway.
E. Nurse assistant applying pressure to a bandage.
F. Nurse assistant giving artificial breaths to a mannequin.

1. ____

2. ____

3. ____

4. ____

5. ____

6. ____

Chapter 13

THEMES OF CARE

Complete each sentence using the correct term.

Autonomy   Maximizing capabilities   Respect   Theme
Infection control   Observation   Safety   Time management

1. A(n) _____ is something repeated over and over.

2. When you work with a resident to their own capabilities, you are _____ .

3. Someone who is able to make decisions for oneself has _____ .

4. _____ involves the use of methods to prevent the transmission of infection.

5. The ability to organize activities and perform them efficiently involves the use of _____ .

6. _____ is the process of watching and paying attention to details.

7. The theme of _____ relates to being free from harm and secure from threats or danger.

8. _____ is to consider worthy of high regard.

ACTIVITY 2 - IDENTIFY THE THEME

Under each example, write the letter of the theme it involves. Some examples require more than one answer. Some themes will be used more than once.

Themes of Care

A. Autonomy
B. Communication
C. Infection control
D. Maximizing capabilities
E. Observation
F. Respect
G. Safety
H. Time management

As you help her dress, you talk with Mrs. Jones about her plans for the day.

1. _____   2. _____

You use gloves as you handle a sputum specimen.

3. _____

You plan ahead, talk with the resident, and organize supplies in advance of any task.

4. _____   5. _____   6. _____

You use a guard belt as you assist Mr. Snodgrass walk down the hallway.

7. _____   8. _____

You encourage Mrs. Fremont to choose what she wears to dinner with her family.

9. _____   10. _____

You dispose of dirty items according to facility policy.

11. _____

Throughout your workday, you make written notes about your residents. Then you use those notes as you do routine reporting.

12. _____   13. _____

Mr. Kent, who is recovering from the flu, asks to choose his clothes and dress himself without any assistance from you. You have noticed that he is stronger, and praise him for doing these things himself.

14. _____   15. _____   16. _____

As you give a.m. care to a resident, you notice that a pipe under the sink is leaking. You clean up the puddle of water, report the problem to the building engineer, and tell staff about it during routine reporting.

17. _____   18. _____

As you help to turn Mrs. Scully in bed, you notice a slight redness on the heel of her right foot. You notify the charge nurse immediately.

19. _____   20. _____

ACTIVITY 3 – MULTIPLE CHOICE

Circle the letter beside the best answer.

1. What is a theme of care?
   A. A special holiday service for residents.
   B. A song that you quietly sing to yourself.
   C. A facility procedure.
   D. A behavior you incorporate into everything you do.

2. Why are the themes of care important?
   A. They make it possible to balance your work time and free time.
   B. When you use them, you will always get your work done early.
   C. They help you balance the art of caregiving and science of nursing.
   D. When you use them, you don't waste as many supplies and clean linens.

3. What is the BEST way to maximize a resident's capabilities?
   A. Allow the resident to do whatever they like.
   B. Make sure residents enjoy their daily personal care routine.
   C. Work with the resident's capabilities and support them to their fullest.
   D. Always do exactly what the family wants you to do for their loved one.

4. What is the BEST way to use time management in your work?
   A. Discourage residents from any changes in their routines.
   B. Try to arrive at work no more than 30 minutes late.
   C. Plan ahead, organize your activities, and perform them efficiently.
   D. Every hour, create a new list of everything you need to do.

5. As a nurse assistant, your task isn't complete until you have:
   A. Put fresh flowers in the room.
   B. Checked the next day's forecast.
   C. Checked the resident's environment.
   D. Smoothed any wrinkles from your uniform.

In the space provided, match each situation to the appropriate response and themes of care.

Situation	Response
1. _____ A co-worker is out sick today and you pick up 3 extra residents to care for. Mrs. Bennet is bedridden and is scheduled for a bath, Mr. Darcy is ambulatory but needs help with bathing, and Mrs. Lucas will need help with buttons and zippers. How can you add these 3 residents to your schedule without compromising the care your other residents receive?	A. Talk to your co-workers about the resident's abilities (communication, observation). If they think the resident is able to bathe alone, allow them to do so with supervision (autonomy, respect, safety).
2. _____ Mr. Wickham is a new resident who wants to do as much as he can for himself. He is scheduled for a tub bath today, and he insists that he can get himself in and out of the tub alone. You have not worked with this resident, but some of your co-workers have. What should you do?	B. Let the charge nurse know that the resident seems sluggish and weak this morning (observation, communication). Ask the nurse for guidance before you assist the resident with walking (maximizing capabilities, safety).
3. _____ Mrs. Collins is recovering from a stroke, which has caused left-sided weakness. You have helped her walk several times this week, but today you had a difficult time getting her out of bed. How should you proceed?	C. Clean up the spill immediately (safety, infection control). Notify the charge nurse and your co-workers that a resident has had an accident (communication). Check each of your residents for signs for incontinence (observation).
4. _____ Mrs. Phillips has mild dementia. She sometimes tastes or touches the food on other residents' trays. What can you do to deal with this problem?	D. Make a plan before you begin giving care (time management). Check to see that none of your residents has an immediate need, such as assistance with toileting (respect, safety). Let them know you will be back to help them with their baths (communication). Schedule the tub room for any residents you will assist with bathing (time management). Assist the more independent residents with dressing (maximizing capabilities). Ask them if they need additional assistance (respect). Assist other residents with their tub bath. Finally, assist your most dependent residents with personal care, such as a bed bath.
5. _____ You notice a puddle of yellow liquid on the floor. You suspect that it may be urine, but you don't know which resident has had an accident. How do you deal with the situation?	E. Ensure that the resident is not hungry by checking their tray after meals (observation). Offer the resident snacks between meals. Try to watch the resident as trays are being passed out, so that you can prevent any problems (observation). When a problem does occur, be sure to replace the item (infection control).

Chapter 14

CREATING A HOME FOR THE RESIDENT

Using the medical terms listed below, complete each sentence correctly.

Axillary
Blood Pressure
Oral

Pulse
Rectal
Relocation stress syndrome

Respiration
Temperature
Tympanic

Vital signs

1. The pressure of blood in the arteries is called _____ .

2. Anxiety in a new resident may be a sign of _____ .

3. _____ temperature is taken in the armpit.

4. The measure of a resident's heart rate is called the _____ .

5. A(n) _____ temperature is taken under the tongue.

6. _____ is another word for breathing.

7. A person's _____ temperature is taken in their eardrum.

8. When you have checked a person's blood pressure, pulse, respirations, and temperature, you have taken their _____

   _____ .

9. _____ temperature is taken in the rectum.

10. The degree of heat that naturally occurs within the body is called _____ .

ACTIVITY 2 – SPELL IT OUT

Using the terms in the box, spell out each word beside the correct description.

Adjustment
Dentures
Deteriorate
Discharge
Mercury
Occupied
Permission
Policy
Protocol
Transfer
Unoccupied

1. A facility's official way of doing something, usually put in writing: ___ R ___ ___ ___ C ___ ___

2. A high level plan for meeting goals, acceptable procedure: ___ ___ L ___ ___ ___

3. The act of giving formal consent: ___ ___ ___ M ___ ___ ___ I ___ ___

4. A bed that is empty: ___ ___ O ___ ___ ___ P ___ ___ ___

5. Process that occurs when a resident is leaving the facility: ___ ___ S ___ ___ ___ ___ ___ E

6. A correction or modification for actual conditions: ___ ___ ___ U ___ ___ ___ N ___

7. To grow worse: ___ ___ T ___ ___ ___ ___ ___ ___ E

8. A heavy silvery poisonous metal that is liquid at ordinary temperatures: ___ ___ R ___ ___ ___ ___

9. Process that occurs when a resident moves from one place to another: ___ ___ ___ N ___ F ___ ___

10. False teeth: ___ E ___ ___ ___ U ___ ___ ___ ___

11. The resident is in the bed: ___ C ___ U ___ ___ ___ ___

ACTIVITY 3 – MATCHING

Match the personnel or department with the role they have in admitting a resident.

Personnel/Department

1. _____ Admission coordinator

2. _____ Dietary department

3. _____ Front office

4. _____ Housekeeping department

5. _____ Maintenance department

6. _____ Nurses

7. _____ Social worker

Role

A. Help the family with financial issues; sometimes may admit new residents.

B. Primary responsibility for admitting a new resident.

C. Clean and set up the room.

D. Help with move in; may set up phone for new resident.

E. Set up payment schedules.

F. Interview residents to find out their food preferences.

G. Start the assessment process; obtain and confirm all doctor's orders.

ACTIVITY 4 – MULTIPLE CHOICE

Circle the letter beside the best answer.

1. Just before placing a thermometer in a resident's mouth, how should you clean it?
   A. Dip it in a strong disinfectant.
   B. Hold it under hot running water.
   C. Wipe it on your sleeve or a clean gown.
   D. Rinse off the disinfectant under cold running water.

2. Mrs. Buckland's pulse is slow every time you check it. What could cause her to have a slow pulse?
   A. Being angry.
   B. Being relaxed.
   C. Being excited.
   D. Recent exercise.

3. Diastolic pressure is a measure of:
   A. Pressure inside a tank of oxygen.
   B. Pressure inside the facility's water heater.
   C. Pressure in the artery when the heart is at rest.
   D. Pressure in the artery when a person is running.

4. What is important when making an occupied bed?
   A. Always roll the resident towards you.
   B. Always roll the resident away from you.
   C. Start at the head of the bed and work down.
   D. Transfer the resident into a chair before you begin.

5. When a resident is transferring into the unit, it is important to:
   A. Treat the resident like a new admission.
   B. Wait for them to come to you with any questions.
   C. Bring them candy or flowers on their first day there.
   D. Ask the administrator to give them a tour of the unit.

ACTIVITY 5 – TRUE/FALSE

Read each statement. Write T in the space provided if the statement is true or F if it is false.

1. _____ A nurse assistant can make a dramatic difference in a new resident's adjustment to the facility.

2. _____ To get the most accurate reading of a person's temperature, you should use the axillary method.

3. _____ A normal pulse rate for an adult at rest is 60 to 90 beats per minute.

4. _____ You should not use your thumb for taking a pulse.

5. _____ A resident's arm should be elevated above the heart when you take a blood pressure reading.

6. _____ A new resident can bring in personal items such as photos, plants, and wall hangings.

7. _____ After a resident has lived at the facility for a week or so, staff no longer needs to knock on their door before entering.

8. _____ A draw sheet is used as a temporary screen when a resident's privacy curtain is being washed.

9. _____ If you find that a call light is not working properly, you should report it immediately.

10. _____ Discharge from a nursing facility is always a happy occasion for a resident and their family.

ACTIVITY 6 – LABELING

A. Correctly read a mercury sphygmomanometer.

1. What is the systolic blood pressure reading? _____

2. What is the diastolic blood pressure reading? _____

B. Correctly read the temperature measured by the glass thermometers shown here.

3. _____

4. _____

ACTIVITY 7 – CONTENT REVIEW

List 5 ways a nurse assistant can help a new resident feel comfortable about being in a nursing facility.

1. _____

2. _____

3. _____

4. _____

5. _____

List 2 fears a resident could have when they are being discharged to a less restrictive setting or home.

6. _____

7. _____

ACTIVITY 8 – LABELING

Using the list provided, label each photo.

A. Nurse assistant taking a resident's oral temperature.
B. Nurse assistant taking an axillary temperature.
C. Nurse assistant taking a resident's pulse.

1. _____

2. _____

3. _____

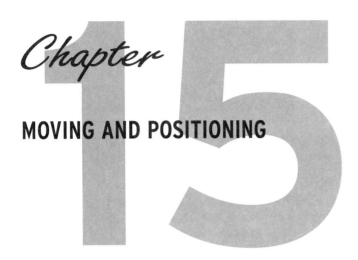

MOVING AND POSITIONING

ACTIVITY 1 – CROSSWORD PUZZLE

Complete the puzzle using the terms and clues provided below.

Adapt
Assess
Fragile
Independent
Intravenous
Limb
Mobility
Osteoporosis
Pivot
Positioning
Supine
Transfer

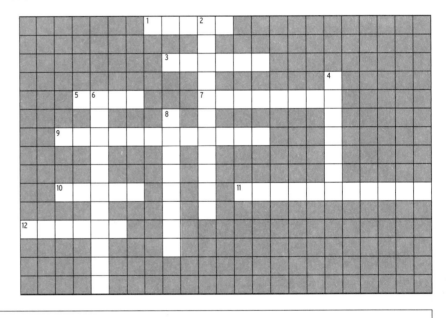

ACROSS

1. change to fit new conditions

3. gather information to make a decision

5. arm or leg

7. move a resident from one surface to another

9. a disease that makes bones porous or chalk-like and very fragile

10. to turn

11. not subject to control by others, not dependent

12. lying on the back

DOWN

2. an act of placing or arranging

4. easily broken or destroyed, delicate

6. fluid or nutrition given from a plastic bag through sterile tubing and a needle inserted into a resident's vein

8. capable of moving or being moved

ACTIVITY 2 – TRUE/FALSE

In the space provided, write T if the statement is true or F if the statement is false.

1. _____ The leading cause of nurse assistant injuries is slips and falls.

2. _____ Osteoporosis can cause bed sores.

3. _____ Someone who has been in bed even for a short time may feel stiff or weak.

4. _____ If you don't know a resident well, you should get help before transferring them.

5. _____ You should never use side rails when moving or positioning a resident.

6. _____ A resident is supine if they are sitting up straight.

7. _____ If you position a wheelchair up against a wall, it does not need to be locked.

8. _____ Postural hypotension causes blood to pool in the brain.

9. _____ It is important to have a resident sit up at the side of the bed before transferring them to a chair.

10. _____ A mechanical lift is used to transfer a resident without the assistance of a co-worker.

ACTIVITY 3 – MULTIPLE CHOICE

Circle the letter beside the best answer.

1. Why is it important to be careful when ambulating a resident who has osteoporosis?
   A. A resident with osteoporosis is prone to weakness.
   B. Residents who have osteoporosis get dizzy very quickly.
   C. Residents with osteoporosis are at risk for breaking bones.
   D. Sometimes blood can pool in their extremities and cause confusion.

2. You are walking Mrs. Reynolds down the hall when she becomes faint and begins to fall. What is the BEST way to prevent her from injuring herself?
   A. Pin her against the wall until a co-worker arrives.
   B. Put both arms around her and drag her to a nearby chair.
   C. Holding on to her guard belt, help her sit down on the floor.
   D. Grab hold of her hair to prevent her head from hitting the floor.

3. You are assisting a co-worker as they move a resident up in a chair. Where will your hands be positioned?
   A. One hand on the guard belt, one under their buttocks.
   B. One hand under the resident's knee, the other under their arm.
   C. One hand on the guard belt, the other hand under the resident's knee.
   D. One hand under the resident's arm, the other hand around the resident's ankle.

4. Mrs. Desmond has a hip fracture. You have reminded her that she shouldn't cross her legs, but she forgets. How can you prevent her from re-injuring her hip?
   A. Transfer her back to the bed.
   B. Put a pillow between her legs.
   C. Suggest she stand instead of sit.
   D. Call her doctor to report the problem.

5. When you position a resident on their back, their legs should normally be positioned:
   A. With a pillow between them.
   B. As close together as possible.
   C. With both legs straight and slightly apart.
   D. With one leg straight and one leg slightly bent.

ACTIVITY 4 – SITUATION/RESPONSE

Read each situation. In the space provided, write the letter of the appropriate response to that situation.

Situation	Response
1. _____ Mrs. Saunders has left sided weakness. You have to transfer her out of a wheelchair onto the toilet.	A. Place a gait belt around her waist. Standing on either side of the resident, have a co-worker assist you by pulling up on the belt with one hand and lifting the resident's knees with the other hand.
2. _____ You notice that Mrs. Walters has slumped down in her chair. She is unable to pull herself back up to a comfortable position.	B. Place her in a side-lying position. Stand on the side to which you will turn her. With a hand on her shoulder and the other on her hip, help her turn toward you. Position her head, neck arms, and legs comfortably.
3. _____ Mr. Hudson has been in bed with the flu for several days. He wants to get up and walk to the bathroom.	C. Place a stool or pillow under her feet so that her knees and hips are at the same height.
4. _____ Mrs. Adamson has been lying on her back for almost 2 hours. You need to reposition her.	D. Position the wheelchair so that her strong side is closest to the toilet. Lock the wheels, raise the footrests, and assist her with a stand pivot transfer.
5. _____ You have transferred Mrs. Adjani from the bed to a chair. She says she is comfortable, but you notice that her feet don't touch the floor.	E. To prevent dizziness, have him roll onto his side and then sit at the edge of the bed with his legs dangling for a few minutes.

ACTIVITY 5 – CONTENT REVIEW

In the column to the left, list 5 effects that could occur if a resident is confined to the bed. In the right column, list the body system that is involved in the effect.

Effect	Body System
1. _____	_____
2. _____	_____
3 _____	_____
4. _____	_____
5. _____	_____

1. Describe what makes life worth living for you.

2. Imagine what it must be like to live in a long term care facility. Describe how you would feel if you were a resident.

3. Make a list of things you would like to continue to do if you were a resident in a long term care facility.

Chapter

PERSONAL CARE

ACTIVITY 1 – MATCHING

Review both lists. In the space provided by each term, write the letter of the correct definition.

1. _____ Anus

2. _____ Aspirate

3. _____ Comatose

4. _____ Foreskin

5. _____ Labia

6. _____ Microorganism

7. _____ Perineal

8. _____ Podiatrist

9. _____ Scrotum

10. _____ Urethra

A. an organism of microscopic size

B. the canal in males and females that carries urine from the bladder; in males it also serves as the duct for sperm

C. the posterior opening of the large intestine

D. physician specializing in the care and treatment of the feet

E. to breathe in or draw in by suction

F. a fold of skin that covers the tip of the penis in an uncircumcised male

G. the external pouch in males that contains the testes

H. someone in a coma

I. area of body between the anus and the posterior part of the external genitals

J. the outer and inner fatty folds bounding the vulva

ACTIVITY 2 – FILL IN THE BLANK

Using the words provided, complete each sentence correctly.

Antiseptic
Corn
Drape
Lather
Objective
Observation
Penis
Personal
Perspiration
Pubic
Stimulate
Subjective
Therapeutic
Tolerate
Uncircumcised
Vagina

1. When something can be observed externally, it is _____.

2. When shaving cream or soap is mixed with water it turns into a foam or troth called _____.

3. The genitals are referred to as the _____ area.

4. A(n) _____ is a substance that reduces the growth or action of microorganisms.

5. If you put up with something or endure it, you _____ it.

6. _____ is a saline fluid secreted by sweat glands.

7. When you cover something up, you _____ it.

8. A penis that has foreskin remaining at the tip is _____.

9. Something is _____ if the person feels it internally. It is the opposite of objective.

10. The word _____ means to arouse a function.

11. A(n) _____ is a local hardening and thickening of epidermis (as on a toe).

12. The word _____ refers to a treatment.

13. The _____ is a canal in a female from the uterus to the external orifice of the genitals.

14. If something is private, or refers to a person's body, it is _____.

15. _____ is the act of recognizing and noting a fact.

16. The _____ is the male organ of urination and copulation.

ACTIVITY 3 – TRUE/FALSE

Read each statement. In the space provided, write T if the statement is true, or F if the statement is false.

1. _____ Observing is a major part of your role as a nurse assistant.

2. _____ It is important for a nurse assistant to report changes to the charge nurse.

3. _____ Some changes in a resident's status are not important.

4. _____ A comatose resident should receive oral care no more than 4 times per day.

5. _____ Flossing is a healthy habit for all residents.

6. _____ Before trimming a resident's facial hair, you should check with the charge nurse.

7. _____ Grooming should always reflect the resident's preferences.

8. _____ It is OK to trim a resident's toenails if they ask you to do so.

ACTIVITY 4 – MULTIPLE CHOICE

Circle the letter beside the best answer.

1. As you provide personal care, you should:
   A. Change your uniform.
   B. Always wear a gown, gloves, and mask.
   C. Protect the resident's dignity and privacy.
   D. Ask the resident's roommate to stay in the room.

2. Why is it important to wear gloves when you provide mouth care?
   A. In case the resident's gums bleed.
   B. The resident may have bad breath.
   C. So you won't have to wash your hands.
   D. In case you get toothpaste on your hands.

3. When is the bath water changed during a bed bath?
   A. Before washing the perineum.
   B. After washing the face and neck.
   C. After washing the feet and hands.
   D. Any time the water gets cold, soapy, or dirty.

4. What is the correct way to wash the female perineal area?
   A. Wash the anus first, then the labia.
   B. Wash the pubic area first, then the anus.
   C. Wash the entire area in a circular motion.
   D. Wash back and forth over the entire area twice.

5. When you are helping to dress a resident with a paralyzed arm you should:
   A. Put the shirt on the weak arm last.
   B. Put the shirt on the weak arm first.
   C. Put the shirt on the arm closest to you.
   D. Put the shirt on the arm farthest from you.

ACTIVITY 5 – SUBJECTIVE/OBJECTIVE

Read each description. Write S if the description is subjective, or O if it is objective.

1. _____ While providing foot care, you notice one of Mrs. Russo's toenails is embedded in the skin.

2. _____ Mrs. Kramer says her gums hurt when she brushes her teeth.

3. _____ A resident seems anxious and upset.

4. _____ Mr. Reynolds has a scrape on his forearm.

5. _____ An oral temperature of 102.6 F.

6. _____ Mr. Dawson said, "I don't want to drink my milk."

7. _____ A resident tells you they are in pain.

8. _____ Mrs. Curtis is holding her head between her hands, rocking back and forth, and crying.

ACTIVITY 6 – SITUATION/RESPONSE

In the space provided by each situation, write the letter of the correct response.

Situation

1. _____ Mrs. Bertram, a blind resident in your care, is going out to lunch with her daughter. She wants to look her best for the outing.

2. _____ You find a red spot on a resident's hip. It doesn't go away.

3. _____ Mrs. Crawford has limited mobility in her left shoulder and needs help getting ready for bed.

4. _____ Mr. Price has a chronic problem with dizziness.

5. _____ Mrs. Rushworth insists on wearing a yellow and orange floral blouse with red and black plaid pants.

Response

A. Help the resident by unzipping their dress. As you put a gown on the resident, put the sleeve on their left arm first.

B. Suggest the resident sit at the side of the bed as you help them dress. Help the resident to put on and take off their shoes and socks.

C. Help the resident choose color-coordinated clothes. Get the clothes out of the closet and help the resident put them on.

D. Allow the resident to choose what they want to wear.

E. Let the charge nurse know about the change in the resident's condition immediately.

Chapter 17

ASSISTING WITH NUTRITION

ACTIVITY 1 – FILL IN THE BLANK

Complete each sentence by adding the correct term.

Dehydration   Hydration   Supplements
Dysphagia   Nutrition   Turgor
Esophagus   Salt

1. _____ can occur if a resident does not have adequate fluid intake.

2. Tight skin that does not "tent" has _____, which is a sign of good hydration.

3. The act of nourishing or being nourished is called _____.

4. Maintaining an adequate fluid level in the body is _____.

5. _____ is also called sodium.

6 Someone who has difficulty chewing or swallowing food has a condition known as _____.

7. The _____ is a muscular tube that leads from the mouth to the stomach.

8. Residents who need additional nutrition may receive it in concentrated amounts through _____.

ACTIVITY 2 – TRUE/FALSE

In the space provided, write T if the statement is true, or F if the statement is false.

1. _____ The food service department provides support with finances.

2. _____ A resident's nutritional status can be enhanced with a combination of correct diet and proper assistance from the nurse assistant.

3. _____ All residents are given a therapeutic diet.

4. _____ A calorie-restricted diet is usually ordered for diabetics.

5. _____ A resident who has difficulty swallowing has aphasia.

6. _____ The food service department uses a feeding tube to mix foods.

7. _____ Intake is the measurement of food and fluids a resident takes in.

8. _____ A nurse assistant measures a resident's weight just to have something to talk about with family members.

9. _____ It is critical to monitor a resident's fluid intake and output.

10. _____ You should notify the charge nurse immediately if a resident's weight drops 1 pound in 2 months.

ACTIVITY 3 – MULTIPLE CHOICE

Circle the letter by the best answer.

1. Why is it important to "liberalize" therapeutic diets?
   A. So that they will be more nutritious.
   B. Therapeutic diets contain too much sugar.
   C. Therapeutic diets are generally too low in calories.
   D. A person may not eat as much if their diet is too restricted.

2. Renal diets often restrict:
   A. Fats.
   B. Fiber.
   C. Sugar.
   D. Protein.

3. As you distribute meals to residents, you should check to see if:
   A. Each tray has a bud vase and flower.
   B. Each meal includes a serving of red meat.
   C. Each tray has the right diet for the resident.
   D. Each meal has only fat-free, sugar-free desserts.

4. What happens when a person aspirates their food?
   A. They feel like taking a nap.
   B. They throw up their dinner.
   C. They feel the need to belch.
   D. They may develop pneumonia.

5. Which of the following signs is an indication of dehydration?
   A. Sunken eyes.
   B. Good skin turgor.
   C. Alzheimer's disease.
   D. Frequent trips to the bathroom.

6. In order to stay hydrated, a resident must:
   A. Avoid sweet foods.
   B. Keep out of the sun.
   C. Drink plenty of fluids.
   D. Bathe or shower each day.

ACTIVITY 4 – CONVERT THE AMOUNTS

Using these formulas, convert the following serving amounts to cc.

1 ounce (oz) = 30 cc
1 cup = 240 cc

1. A 4 oz serving of orange juice = _____ cc.

2. A 6 oz serving of coffee = _____ cc.

3. A 1/2 cup of Jell-O = _____ cc.

4. A tumbler containing 1 1/2 cups of iced tea = _____ cc.

5. A 3 oz serving of ice cream = _____ cc.

6. An 8 oz bowl of soup = _____ cc.

ACTIVITY 5 – SITUATION/RESPONSE

Match the situation with the appropriate response by a nurse assistant. Some responses will be used more than once.

Situation	Response
1. _____ A resident tells you they cannot cut their meat.	A. Assist the resident.
2. _____ You check a resident's water pitcher and find that it is full.	B. Report this to the charge nurse.
3. _____ A resident ate only 25% of their meal.	C. Obtain the missing item.
4. _____ You pass trays out to residents.	D. Offer the resident water.
5. _____ A resident tells you they are thirsty.	E. Check the tray card and the resident's ID band.
6. _____ A resident cannot open their milk carton.	
7. _____ A tray arrives without utensils.	
8. _____ You are serving a new resident.	
9. _____ A resident says they have the wrong tray.	
10. _____ A resident refuses to eat anything you offer.	

ACTIVITY 6 – LABELING

Identify the percentage of food eaten. Write the letter of the correct percentage by the correct photo.

A. 75%   B. 90%   C. 25%   D. 50%

1. _____

2. _____

3. _____

4. _____

ACTIVITY 7 – CONTENT REVIEW

Write the answers in the space provided. Refer to the textbook if necessary.

Why would residents be placed on the following diets?

1. Calorie-restricted diet:

2. Sodium-restricted diet:

3. Fat/cholesterol-restricted diet:

4. Protein-restricted diet:

5. Why would a resident need supplements?

6. What is your role as a nurse assistant in assisting residents with meals?

Chapter 18

ASSISTING WITH ELIMINATION

ACTIVITY 1 – CROSSWORD PUZZLE

Using the list of terms and the clues provided below, complete the puzzle.

Bladder	Gastrointestinal	Occult	Stoma	Urine
Bowel	Guiacing	Ostomy	Stool	Void
Elimination	Incontinence	Parasite	Urinate	

ACROSS

5. related to the stomach and intestines
7. refers to the large and small intestines
8. an organism that lives in or on another organism
10. the process of ridding the body of urine and stool
11. a surgical opening from the intestine to outside the body
12. waste liquid secreted by the kidney
13. a surgically created opening

DOWN

1. procedure for checking for blood in the stool
2. inability to hold urine or stool is called
3. to eliminate liquid waste from the body
4. sac inside the body that holds urine
6. human waste, or feces, from the bowel
9. to pass urine
11. refers to blood that is present in stool but cannot be seen

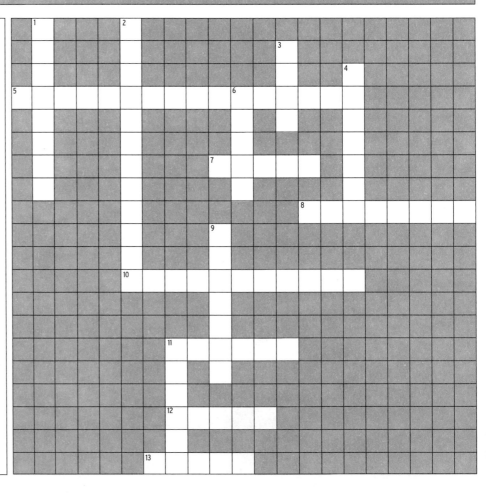

ACTIVITY 2 – FILL IN THE BLANK

Complete each sentence with the correct word.

Analyze   Commode   Concentrated   Frequency

1. A portable toilet, also called a(n) _____ ,
   is a box-like structure with a chamber pot under an open seat.

2. Urine is _____ if it is less diluted, or
   more intense in color.

3. Lab tests are done to _____ the chemical
   parts of urine, stool, or other specimens.

4. _____ refers to how often something
   happens, or a habitual pattern.

ACTIVITY 3 – MULTIPLE CHOICE

Circle the letter beside the best answer.

1. When should you question a new resident about their elimination
   patterns?
   A. While family members are present.
   B. Within minutes after they are admitted.
   C. As you introduce them to other residents.
   D. At a convenient time and in a private place.

2. Solid waste discharged from the bowel is called:
   A. Feces.
   B. Urine.
   C. Stoma.
   D. Guiacing.

3. All specimens are considered to be:
   A. Dirty.
   B. Bloody.
   C. Watery.
   D. Cloudy.

4. When is a clean-catch urine specimen collected?
   A. After a 24-hour fasting period.
   B. After the urethral opening is cleansed.
   C. After the resident has emptied their bladder.
   D. After the resident has had a bowel movement.

5. An ostomy that routes the colon to an opening on the surface of the
   abdomen is called:
   A. A stoma.
   B. A colostomy.
   C. An ileostomy.
   D. A ureterostomy.

ACTIVITY 4 – CONTENT REVIEW

List 3 ways you can determine a resident's elimination pattern.

1. _____

2. _____

3. _____

Describe 4 ways you can help ensure that a resident's elimination pattern stays normal.

4. _____

5. _____

6. _____

7. _____

List 4 ways to help maintain a resident's dignity when assisting them with elimination.

8. _____

9. _____

10. _____

11. _____

ACTIVITY 5 – YES OR NO

For each situation, write Y for yes if it should be reported to the charge nurse, or N for no if you would not report it.

1. _____ The resident's urine had a foul odor.

2. _____ The resident had a painful, hard, black stool today.

3. _____ The resident complained of painful urination.

4. _____ The resident's stool had red blood in it.

5. _____ The resident urinated 2 times during your shift.

6. _____ The resident was incontinent for the first time.

7. _____ The resident drank 2 cups of coffee during your shift.

8. _____ The resident's abdomen is swollen and they have not had a bowel movement in 2 days.

9. _____ The resident's urine was clear.

10. _____ The resident had a watery, foul-smelling stool today.

ACTIVITY 6 – DIGNITY CHECKLIST

Read each statement and indicate if the nurse assistant protected the resident's dignity. In the space provided, write D if the resident's dignity is protected or N if it is not protected.

1. _____ You respond to a resident's call light immediately.

2. _____ You close the door before helping the resident use a bedpan.

3. _____ You tease the resident about wetting herself.

4. _____ You discuss a resident's bowel problems in front of their roommate's family.

5. _____ You left the resident sitting on the toilet for 30 minutes.

6. _____ You talk in private with a resident about their elimination pattern.

7. _____ You leave a stool sample on the desk, with the resident's name clearly marked on the label.

ACTIVITY 7 – LABELING

Match each photo with the name of the item. In the space provided, write the letter found next to the photo.

A. Urinal   B. Bedside commode   C. Fracture pan   D. Bedpan

1. _____

2. _____

3. _____

4. _____

RESTORATIVE ACTIVITIES

ACTIVITY 1 – MATCHING

In the space provided, write the letter of the correct definition for each term.

1. _____ Brace

2. _____ Extremity

3. _____ Orthotic device

4. _____ Prosthetic device

5. _____ Restorative

6. _____ Splint

7. _____ Trapeze

A. device that supports and strengthens a body part

B. supportive equipment made for a resident, such as a brace or splint that supports a limb

C. a limb of the body

D. device made to replace a missing body part or function

E. the process of restoring to a former state

F. device to use to support or immobilize a body part

G. a short horizontal bar suspended by two parallel ropes, used to pull oneself up in bed

ACTIVITY 2 – FILL IN THE BLANK

Using the terms provided below, complete each sentence correctly.

Alert   Function   Optimal
Artificial limb   Immobilized   Prompting
Capability   Independence   Regain
Cuing   Maintain   Stump

1. The portion of an extremity remaining after the rest is removed is called the _____.

2. In order to keep something in its existing state, it is necessary to _____ it.

3. Restorative activities are done in a way to help restore _____, or the action for which a body part is used.

4. If someone is quick to perceive and act on a situation, they are _____.

5. When you give a resident a signal to begin a specific speech or action, you are _____.

6. Moving a person to take an action, or helping them remember something is called _____.

7. In order to prevent freedom of movement, a joint or body part must be _____.

8. The goal of restorative activities is to help a resident achieve their most desirable, or _____, level of functioning.

9. An arm or leg that is human-made is called a(n) _____.

10. _____ refers to a person's ability to do something.

11. A person who is not subject to control by others has _____.

12. Restorative activities can help a person _____ lost function again.

ACTIVITY 3 – MULTIPLE CHOICE

Circle the letter beside the best answer.

1. You are working with a resident who recently had a stroke. It takes the resident a long time to dress himself. How can you help him regain lost function?
   A. Insist on doing everything for him.
   B. Tell the family to help him every day.
   C. Help him so that he gets dressed faster.
   D. Be patient and let him do as much as he can.

2. The nurse asks you to give range-of-motion exercise to Mrs. White, who is confined to bed. According to her care plan, there are no restrictions. What does "no restrictions" mean?
   A. You should work her joints and muscles very hard.
   B. Provide ROM exercise as often as possible on each shift.
   C. Mrs. White should be able to do all of the exercises herself.
   D. You may move each joint through its full available range.

3. Mrs. Wilson seems puzzled or confused when you tell her you'd like her to practice using a walker. How can you help her understand?
   A. Tell her you are in a hurry.
   B. Repeat the request in a different way.
   C. Use baby talk to get your point across.
   D. Tell the next shift nurse assistant to try it.

4. Which of the following is an orthotic device?
   A. Walker
   B. Trapeze
   C. Leg brace
   D. Artificial leg

5. You are about to help Mrs. Paulsen take a walk. She is on oxygen. What is the BEST way to ensure her safety?
   A. Have her take a few deep breaths before you walk.
   B. Carry her oxygen tank under your arm as you walk.
   C. Take her off oxygen for the short time she is walking.
   D. Ask another staff to follow and pull a portable oxygen tank.

ACTIVITY 4 – INDEPENDENT/DEPENDENT

Read the following sentences. In the space provided, write I if the action promotes independence or D if it promotes dependence.

1. _____ A resident wants to walk to the dining room, but you tell him you can get him there quicker by pushing him in a wheelchair.

2. _____ You give a resident a bed bath even though with assistance they could take a shower.

3. _____ You encourage a resident to take a walk while you make the bed.

4. _____ You wheel a resident to the activities room.

5. _____ You encourage a resident to use his cane to take a walk.

6. _____ You say to a resident, "I'll start buttoning your shirt, and you can finish it."

7. _____ A resident can walk a little, but you use a wheelchair all the time.

8. _____ A resident picks up a spoon to eat, but because they are slow you take the spoon and begin feeding them.

9. _____ You hand a piece of bread to a resident who is recovering from a stroke, encouraging them to use their weak hand.

10. _____ You discuss a resident's eating limitations with the charge nurse in hopes of coming up with some assistive devices so they can eat without your help.

ACTIVITY 5 – CONTENT REVIEW

List 2 examples in each category of equipment. Refer to your textbook if necessary.

Assistive devices

1. _____

2. _____

Prosthetic and orthotic devices

1. _____

2. _____

Positioning devices

1. _____

2. _____

Aids for activities of daily living

1. _____

2. _____

ACTIVITY 6 – TRUE/FALSE

Read the following sentences. In the space provided, write T if the statement is true or F if the statement is false.

1. _____ A contracture occurs when a joint becomes stuck in a certain position.

2. _____ Once the interdisciplinary team sets goals for a resident, those goals never change.

3. _____ A disability is a physical problem only and never affects a resident's psychological state.

4. _____ Prompting and cuing are forms of sign language used only to communicate with hearing impaired individuals.

5. _____ One goal of restorative activities is to enable a resident to perform activities of daily living independently.

6. _____ An entire ROM exercise program always takes about 60 minutes.

7. _____ You perform finger flexion when you bend the fingers at each of the joints.

8. _____ Each range of motion exercise should be repeated 5 to 10 times, depending on the resident's comfort level.

ACTIVITY 7 – CONTENT REVIEW

List 2 examples of short- and long-term goals the following residents undergoing rehabilitation might try to achieve. Refer to your textbook if necessary.

Resident 1

Mrs. Hildebrand is recovering from total hip replacement surgery. She is able to sit up on the side of the bed.

1. Short-term goal:

_____

_____

2. Long-term goal:

_____

_____

Resident 2

Mr. Scott recently had a leg amputated below the knee. He has just received his prosthetic leg and is receiving physical therapy each day.

3. Short-term goal:

_____

_____

4. Long-term goal:

_____

_____

Chapter 20

MAINTAINING SKIN INTEGRITY

ACTIVITY 1 – TRUE/FALSE

Write T if the statement is true or F if it is false.

1. _____ Even if a person is born with healthy skin, they are at risk for pressure ulcers when they are elderly.

2. _____ Only a nurse or doctor can identify redness on the skin.

3. _____ An overweight person can't develop pressure ulcers.

4. _____ ROM exercises can improve circulation.

5. _____ As a nurse assistant, you are in the best position to observe the resident's skin from head to toe.

6. _____ Daily inspection of the skin is an excellent way to prevent pressure ulcers.

7. _____ Stage IV pressure ulcers should be treated only with daily bathing.

8. _____ A resident is at high risk for skin breakdown if they cannot go to the toilet by themselves.

9. _____ Stage I pressure ulcers have a foul smell or discharge.

10. _____ Active people are at greater risk for skin breakdown.

11. _____ Cornstarch should be applied to a stage III decubitus ulcer.

12. _____ Adequate nutrition and fluid intake are required for healthy skin.

13. _____ Bed sore is another term for decubitus ulcer.

14. _____ If you think a change in a resident's skin isn't serious, then you don't need to report it.

15. _____ Shearing force can occur when you slide a resident across their bed.

ACTIVITY 2 – MATCHING

Match the nurse assistant's task with the preventative strategy.

Condition	Preventative Strategy
1. ____ Helping an immobile resident maintain good circulation.	A. Mobility
2. ____ Being attentive to any changes in the resident's skin condition.	B. Nutrition
3. ____ Encouraging a resident to eat their meals.	C. Observation
4. ____ Helping an incontinent resident to stay clean and dry.	D. Range-of-motion (ROM) exercise
5. ____ Assisting a resident to ambulate.	E. Bathing/moisturizing
6. ____ Telling the charge nurse about changes to a resident's skin.	F. Reporting

ACTIVITY 3 – MULTIPLE CHOICE

Circle the letter beside the best answer.

1. Skin that has integrity is:
   A. Tanned, tough, and thick.
   B. Free of moles or birth marks.
   C. Free of cuts, bruises, or wounds.
   D. Only found on babies and children.

2. What is a decubitus ulcer?
   A. A stomach ulcer that is caused by stress.
   B. An ulcer appearing only in people with AIDS.
   C. A wound that appears in pressure areas of the skin.
   D. An ulcer of the lips or mouth that is caused by a virus.

3. Shearing occurs when:
   A. You tear a sheet as you are making a bed.
   B. You put too much alcohol on a razor burn.
   C. Skin rubs against an object or another area of skin.
   D. A resident's skin remains damp for hours at a time.

4. Circulation of blood to the skin is enhanced by:
   A. Eating.
   B. Talking.
   C. Walking.
   D. Sleeping.

5. You can help maintain a resident's skin by:
   A. Inspecting it carefully every day.
   B. Taking them outside on sunny days.
   C. Giving them a daily dose of caster oil.
   D. Rubbing it hourly with antibiotic ointment.

ACTIVITY 4 – SITUATION/RESPONSE

Match the situation with the correct response.

Situation	Response
1. _____ Mrs. Leamus has thin, delicate skin. You notice that her thighs tend to stick to the toilet seat.	A. Encourage the resident to eat all their meals and drink plenty of fluids. Inspect the resident's skin daily. Be sure the bed linens are free of wrinkles before the resident goes to sleep.
2. _____ Mr. Mundt has a scratch on his elbow. It was caused by rough spot on the arm rest of his wheelchair.	B. Follow the charge nurse's instructions for treatment of the problem. Check frequently to see that the resident's heel is not resting on the bed.
3. _____ Mrs. Guillam is confined to bed. She is being treated for a stage II decubitus ulcer on her right heel.	C. Assist resident to the toilet on a frequent basis. When the resident wets themselves, clean their perineal area with soap and water before putting on a clean incontinence brief.
4. _____ Mrs. Crail is confused, underweight, and has little interest in food. When she sleeps, she tends to thrash around in bed, pulling at the sheets and covers.	D. Inspect the resident's thighs for skin breakdown. Use cornstarch on the toilet seat to prevent shearing. Notify the charge nurse about the situation.
5. _____ Mr. Karden is incontinent and wears an incontinence brief.	E. Ask the charge nurse what to do about the scratch. Place a pillow between the resident's arm and the arm rest until the rough spot can be removed from the arm rest.

ACTIVITY 5 – IN YOUR OWN WORDS

1. Describe what makes life worth living for you.

2. Imagine what it must be like to live in a long term care facility. Describe how you would feel if you were a resident.

3. Make a list of things you would like to continue to do if you were a resident in a long term care facility.

Chapter 21

PAIN MANAGEMENT, SLEEP, AND COMFORT

ACTIVITY 1 – SPELL IT OUT

Using the definitions and clues provided, finish spelling out each word.

Acupuncture
Distraction
Endorphins
Guided imagery
Pain

1. These are natural morphine-like substances released by the brain during exercise, which can alter pain sensation:
   _ _ _ _ D _ _ _ _ N _

2. A bodily sensation that causes suffering and distress: _ _ _ _ N

3. This technique is used to direct a person's attention away from their pain or discomfort: _ _ _ _ _ T _ _ _ _ _ _ _ _ _ N

4. This is a medical therapy that originated in ancient China: _ C _ _ _ _ _ _ _ T _ _ _ _

5. Relaxation can be achieved through this technique involving words and music: _ U _ _ _ _ _ _ I _ _ _ _ R _

ACTIVITY 2 – TRUE/FALSE

Read each statement. In the space provided, write T if the statement is true and F if the statement is false.

1. _____ Untreated pain can cause a decline in a resident's health.

2. _____ A nurse assistant has an important role in helping a resident who has pain.

3. _____ Most types of pain are a normal part of aging.

4. _____ If a resident can smile, they are not in pain.

5. _____ Unmanaged pain can cause a person to feel depressed, anxious, and fearful.

6. _____ Hot applications are used to reduce swelling 24 hours after an injury.

7. _____ Cold applications can help to control bleeding.

8. _____ Unpleasant odors can prevent a resident from sleeping.

9. _____ Pain is the fifth vital sign.

10. _____ Residents have a right to have their pain treated.

ACTIVITY 3 – MATCHING

Match the misconception about pain with the fact.

Misconception	Fact
1. _____ It is better not to take pain medicine until the pain is really bad.	A. People can develop a tolerance to medication. It does not mean they are addicted or immune. They just need a stronger dose or a new medication.
2. _____ It is easier to deal with pain than the side effects of pain medication.	B. The risk of addiction is rare when the medication is taken for pain.
3. _____ If a resident takes too much pain medication, they will become addicted.	C. If you wait too long to take pain medicine, you may need a higher dose or stronger medicine. Taking medicine regularly can help prevent pain.
4. _____ Pain is a normal part of aging.	D. Pain happens more frequently for older people, but it is not normal and should be treated.
5. _____ If pain medicine no longer works for a resident, they must be addicted or immune to it.	E. It is important to treat pain. The nursing staff wants to help a resident who is in pain.
6. _____ Nurses and nurse assistants are too busy to be bothered about a resident's pain.	F. Pain medicines can cause side effects, but the side effects are treatable. Worries about side effects should not stop someone from taking pain medicine.

ACTIVITY 4 – MULTIPLE CHOICE

Circle the letter of the best answer.

1. What is the nurse assistant's role in helping residents who are in pain?
   A. To always offer the resident a hot compress for their pain.
   B. To always lead a resident through a guided imagery exercise.
   C. To always tell the charge nurse whenever a resident is in pain.
   D. To always notify the family whenever their loved one is in pain.

2. If a resident tells you their pain is a 3 on a scale of 10, what should you do?
   A. You should offer them an aspirin.
   B. You should tell the charge nurse promptly.
   C. You shouldn't do anything for so little pain.
   D. You should tell them not to worry until it is 8 or 9.

3. Untreated pain can cause a resident to feel:
   A. Sleepy.
   B. Hungry.
   C. Healthy.
   D. Hopeless.

4. A sitz bath is a type of:
   A. Dry cold.
   B. Moist heat.
   C. Acupuncture.
   D. Guided imagery.

5. What is a common side effect of pain medication?
   A. Swelling.
   B. Itchy skin.
   C. Incontinence.
   D. Constipation.

ACTIVITY 5 – MATCHING

Match the letter of the correct description to the non-drug therapy.

Non-drug therapy	Description
1. _____ Acupuncture	A. A technique that uses words and sometimes music to achieve a relaxed and focused state.
2. _____ Animals	B. Strategies to reduce anxiety, muscle tension, and pain that include meditation and deep breathing.
3. _____ Distraction	C. Laughter is used as a form of distraction.
4. _____ Guided imagery	D. Pet therapy programs provide relaxation and companionship as a form of distraction.
5. _____ Heat/cold application	E. A form of electrical massage applied to specific areas of the body.
6. _____ Humor	F. A healing method in which fine needles are inserted in the body at certain sites.
7. _____ Massage	G. This application is used in various dry or moist forms to relieve pain or increase comfort.
8. _____ Relaxation	H. A form of relaxation that involves the use of slow rhythmic strokes on specific areas of the body.
9. _____ Vibration	I. Technique in which the goal is to focus the resident's attention on something other than their pain.

ACTIVITY 6 – SITUATION/RESPONSE

Match each situation with the action a nurse assistant should take.

Situation	Response
1. _____ The charge nurse has applied a hot water bottle to a resident's hip to relieve pain.	A. Let the charge nurse know. It may be necessary for the resident to receive a laxative or stool softener.
2. _____ You notice Mrs. Carlton is rubbing her shoulder and grimacing. You ask her if she is in pain and she says "No."	B. Assure her that the nurse wants to know whenever a resident is in pain. Tell the charge nurse about the resident's pain.
3. _____ You notice that a resident seems to be in pain. You ask her about it, but she says she doesn't want to bother the nurse for medication.	C. Tell the charge nurse what you've observed and what the resident told you.
4. _____ You notice that a resident who is on pain medication has not had a bowel movement in 2 days.	D. Tell the charge nurse what you've noticed. Extra sleep may be a sign of over-medication.
5. _____ Mr. Acton has been on pain medication for 3 days. He has begun to sleep for several hours in the afternoon.	E. Follow the charge nurse's instructions. Check with the resident every 5 to 10 minutes. Check the site for signs of redness.

1. Describe what makes life worth living for you.

2. Imagine what it must be like to live in a long term care facility. Describe how you would feel if you were a resident.

3. Make a list of things you would like to continue to do if you were a resident in a long term care facility.

CARE OF RESIDENTS WITH ALZHEIMER'S DISEASE AND RELATED DISORDERS

Using the list of terms, complete each sentence correctly.

Agenda behavior   Behavioral symptoms   Hallucination   Wandering
Agitation   Cognitive impairment   Insomnia   Sundown syndrome
Alzheimer's disease   Delusion   Multi-infarct
Anxiety   Dementia   Symptoms

1. A false thought that is thought to be real is called a(n) _____.

2. _____ is a progressive, incurable disease that affects the brain and causes memory loss and eventual death.

3. _____ are subjective evidence of disease or condition.

4. When a resident tends to follow a certain agenda, often a past routine, their behavior is referred to as _____.

5. A resident's movements that are irregular, rapid, violent, or excited and often troubled suggest the resident is experiencing

    _____.

6. Actions that are caused by a disease or condition are known as _____.

7. When a person moves from one place to another aimlessly, they are _____.

8. _____ is a situation later in the day when a resident may become irritable or combative, or tearful and withdrawn.

9. When a person cannot sleep enough, they have _____.

10. _____ means that a person is experiencing a disruption in knowledge, memory, awareness, or judgment.

11. The term _____ refers to a loss of mental functions such as memory, thinking, and reasoning.

12. A person is having a(n) _____ when they see or hear things that are not really there.

13. _____ is a state of uneasiness in the mind.

14. _____ is a type of damage to blood vessels that may cause a loss of function in a tissue or organ, such as the brain.

ACTIVITY 2 – SPELL IT OUT

Using the clues and terms provided, complete the spelling of each word.

Confront   Distraction   Maximize   Technique   Validation

1. To increase something to the maximum: : _ _ _ _ _ M _ _ _ _

2. To face someone with a challenge: _ _ _ _ F _ _ _ _

3. Confirmation of something: _ _ _ _ _ D _ _ _ _ N

4. A method for reaching a desired goal: _ _ C _ _ _ _ _ _ E

5. Something that distracts the resident's attention or eases mental confusion: _ _ S _ R _ _ _ _ _ _

ACTIVITY 3 – MULTIPLE CHOICE

Circle the best answer to each question.

1. Alzheimer's disease is a form of:
   A. Cancer.
   B. Dementia.
   C. Osteoporosis.
   D. Cerebral palsy.

2. How can you prevent a resident who has dementia from becoming agitated?
   A. Confine the resident to their room.
   B. Provide a quiet, controlled environment.
   C. Repeatedly tell the resident to stay calm.
   D. Provide lots of exciting large group activities.

3. Mrs. Dodson says everyone wants to steal her things. This suggests she is:
   A. Delusional.
   B. Short of breath.
   C. Hard of hearing.
   D. Just teasing the staff.

4. One of your responsibilities in caring for residents with dementia is to:
   A. Anticipate their basic needs.
   B. Give them presents on holidays.
   C. Hide them from family members.
   D. Prevent them from taking too much of your time.

5. Mr. Smith tells you he has to go to work today. Using the technique called validation therapy, how would you respond to his demand to go to work?
   A. Tell him that he is too old and sick to work.
   B. Ignore his continued requests for your attention.
   C. Tell him today is a holiday and he doesn't have to work.
   D. Remind him that he is retired and has Alzheimer's disease.

ACTIVITY 4 – MATCHING

Match each behavioral term with the example of that behavior and an approach to care.

1. _____ Mr. Alvin doesn't do crossword puzzles anymore and always seems sad and tired. You encourage him to talk about how he feels.

2. _____ Mr. Hendricks taps his foot on the floor repeatedly. You make sure there is no physical problem causing his distress.

3. _____ Mrs. Penrose has an increased pulse rate and appears tense. You assure her that she is safe.

4. _____ Mrs. Rushman never sleeps more than 2 hours a night. You help her to eat properly and rest during the day.

5. _____ Mrs. Wiley believes that her family wants to hurt her. You help her feel loved and supported, without arguing about her beliefs.

6. _____ Mr. Randall sometimes has conversations with people who are not there. You listen to him without questioning who he is talking to.

7. _____ Mr. Williamson walks up and down the hallway, opening and closing doors. You help him get routine exercise.

A. Agitation

B. Anxiety

C. Delusions

D. Depression

E. Hallucinations

F. Insomnia

G. Wandering

ACTIVITY 5 – RESPONSIBILITY REVIEW

List the 6 principles that guide your activities when caring for residents with Alzheimer's disease. Refer to your textbook as needed to complete this exercise. Hint: one principle is to "Provide Guidance and Direction."

1a. _____

2a. _____

3a. _____

4a. _____

5a. _____

6a. _____

List the 6 techniques that will help you support the resident and lessen the intensity of some behavioral symptoms. Refer to your textbook as needed to complete this exercise. Hint: one technique is to "Enter a Resident's Reality."

1b. _____

2b. _____

3b. _____

4b _____

5b. _____

6b. _____

ACTIVITY 6 – MATCHING

Match the factors that cause resistance to care with the description of that factor.

Factor	Description
1. ___ Medical/emotional factors	A. Responding to your negative body language, tone of voice, or facial expressions.
2. ___ Communication factors	B. Unmet basic needs such as hunger, thirst, pain or the need for elimination.
3. ___ Environmental factors	C. The resident's needs change as the disease progresses.
4. ___ Nature of the task	D. The resident may not understand the procedure or what is expected of them.
5. ___ Stage of the disease	E. The room may be too cold, too dark, have too much equipment, etc.

ACTIVITY 7 – STRATEGY REVIEW

Describe a strategy you can use to overcome resistance caused by each of these factors listed in Activity 6.

1. Medical/emotional factors:

   _____

   _____

2. Communication factors:

   _____

   _____

3. Environmental factors:

   _____

   _____

4. Nature of the task:

   _____

   _____

5. Stage of the disease:

   _____

   _____

ACTIVITY 8 – CONTENT REVIEW

For each activity of daily living listed below, write 2 guidelines you can use to assist a resident who has dementia. Refer to your textbook as needed to complete this exercise.

Toileting

1. _____

2. _____

Hydration

3. _____

4. _____

Eating

5 _____

6. _____

Dressing

7. _____

8. _____

Bathing

9. _____

10. _____

Grooming

11. _____

12. _____

Refer to the textbook as needed to complete each exercise or answer each question.

1. Have you ever thought to yourself, "I can't absorb any more information. My head is spinning"? What do you do in situations like this?

2. What do you think it is like to feel overwhelmed every moment of your life?

3. How would you want the people around you to behave when you are feeling overwhelmed?

OTHER RESIDENT POPULATIONS

ACTIVITY 1 – FILL IN THE BLANK

Using the terms provided below, complete each sentence correctly.

Adaptive skills   Developmental disability   Habilitation model   Mental retardation
Autism   Down syndrome   Individual service plan   Normalization
Cerebral palsy   Epilepsy   IQ test

1. A philosophy of care in which an individual with a developmental disability is educated or trained to participate as fully as possible in all aspects of life, including interaction with their family and community, and to have a satisfying social life, is called the

   _____ _____ .

2. _____ is a rare, severe disorder in which the child withdraws from the world; the cause is not known, and there is no cure.

3. Damage to the central nervous system before, during, or after birth can cause _____ _____ .

4. An individual program plan, also known as _____ _____ ,
   is a plan of care that provides special accommodations and sets the priorities of care for the resident.

5. _____ is a disorder of the nervous system that causes seizures and may cause a developmental disability.

6. A(n) _____ is a measure of a person's intelligence.

7. People use _____ _____ everyday to live, work, and play.

8. A(n) _____ _____ is a chronic, severe condition that a person develops from any of many causes, which prevents them from living independently without assistance.

9. _____ _____ is a condition in which a person is born with an extra chromosome, causing some level of mental retardation, abnormal features, and often other medical problems; also known as mongolism and trisomy 21 syndrome.

10. An individual has _____ _____ when they have significantly below-average intelligence and minimal adaptive skills.

11. The creation of an environment for individuals with developmental disabilities that is as close to normal as possible is called

   _____ .

ACTIVITY 2 – MULTIPLE CHOICE

Circle the letter of the best answer.

1. Assisted living facilities are also known as:
   A. Subacute care facilities.
   B. Residential care facilities.
   C. Inpatient recovery centers.
   D. Radiation treatment centers.

2. What is a typical example of a person in a subacute care unit?
   A. A person who has mental retardation.
   B. A person suffering from chicken pox or measles.
   C. A person with a severe developmental disability.
   D. A person who has had knee replacement surgery.

3. Which of these conditions is always present before birth?
   A. Autism.
   B. Epilepsy.
   C. Down syndrome.
   D. Mental retardation.

4. What is fragile X syndrome?
   A. A mild infection.
   B. A genetic disorder.
   C. Fetal alcohol syndrome.
   D. A virus that causes fragile bones.

5. What is another name for an individual habilitation plan?
   A. Annual progress report.
   B. Individual program plan.
   C. Interdisciplinary care plan.
   D. Normalization status report.

ACTIVITY 3 – TRUE/FALSE

In the space provided, write T for true or F for false.

1. _____ Autism can be cured by antibiotics.

2. _____ Most people use their adaptive skills everyday.

3. _____ The typical stay in a subacute care facility is less than 30 days.

4. _____ Residents in assisted living facilities must cook their own meals.

5. _____ The abbreviation "IQ" means intelligence quotient.

6. _____ People with epilepsy are rarely able to hold jobs.

7. _____ Cerebral palsy can occur after birth.

8. _____ A person who has Down syndrome is missing an extremity.

9. _____ You can always tell a person has HIV by the way they look.

10. _____ A resident of an ICF/MR must be over the age of 18.

ACTIVITY 4 – CONTENT REVIEW

Read each description below. In the space provided, write the name of the disease or disability that applies.

Autism
Cerebral palsy
Down syndrome
Epilepsy
HIV/AIDS
Mental retardation

Mr. Wilkins is 28 years old and lives in a group home. He is short and his face is noticeable because of his slanted eyes and protruding tongue. He is able to communicate, bathe, dress, and feed himself. He is not able to hold a job or attend a regular school.

1. _____

Betsy is 10 years old and has frequent convulsions. She is on medication to control the convulsions, but must live in a facility where her condition can be controlled. She attends a special school.

2. _____

Teddy is 8 years old, and has a normal appearance. He does not respond to the people around him and does not liked to be touched. He sometimes bangs his head against the wall and chants words or phrases over and over. He lives in a group home and requires constant supervision.

3. _____

Mr. Dickenson is 36 years old and lives in a group home. He lacks the intelligence needed to take care of his basic needs. He cannot leave the facility without supervision and assistance.

4. _____

Janie is 14 years old and lives in a facility for the developmentally disabled. She has mild paralysis in her arms and legs and spends her days in a special wheelchair. She talks with great difficulty and sometimes has seizures. She receives ROM exercises daily.

5. _____

Mr. Russo is a former drug abuser who lives in a nursing facility. He is underweight and suffers from skin rashes, diarrhea, and fatigue. He frequently has a fever. His disease has no cure.

6. _____

ACTIVITY 5 – CRITICAL THINKING

1. Think about working in the settings that have been described in this chapter. Based on what you have learned, describe how caregiving would be different in each of these types of facilities. How would you adapt your care?

Assisted Living Facility

_____

_____

_____

Subacute Care Unit

_____

_____

_____

ICF/MR

_____

_____

_____

HIV/AIDS Unit

_____

_____

_____

Chapter

END OF LIFE

ACTIVITY 1 – MATCHING

Write the letter of the correct definition in the space provided by each term.

Term	Definition
1. _____ Bereavement	A. Care focused on comfort and symptom relief rather than cure
2. _____ Hospice	B. Rebirth in another form of life
3. _____ Living will/advanced directive	C. A program with a specially trained interdisciplinary team that cares for a terminally ill resident expected to die within 6 months
4. _____ Palliative	D. Period of grief after a loved one dies
5. _____ Reincarnation	E. A legal document used by a resident to communicate their wishes about the care they want if they become incapacitated and cannot make decisions

ACTIVITY 2 – MULTIPLE CHOICE

Circle the letter next to the best answer.

1. You can help a dying resident cope with their feelings by:
   A. Avoiding painful topics.
   B. Forcing them to face reality.
   C. Sharing your own views about death.
   D. Listening to anything they have to say.

2. What is an advance directive?
   A. A last will and testament that is signed before the age of 50.
   B. A signed document which outlines a person's plan for reincarnation.
   C. A legal document stating the person's wishes about lifesaving care or death.
   D. A legal document stating what is to be done with your belongings after your death.

3. When a dying resident voices their anger, what should you say?
   A. "You shouldn't feel that way."
   B. "Everybody goes through this stage."
   C. "What you're going through is really hard, isn't it?"
   D. "Would you please try not to take your anger out on me?"

4. You can help the family of a dying resident by:
   A. Insisting that they pray with you.
   B. Telling them jokes or amusing stories.
   C. Helping them to laugh about their troubles.
   D. Being available to listen when they want to talk.

5. When a resident wants to talk about their funeral arrangements, it usually means they've reached the stage of:
   A. Resolution.
   B. Bargaining.
   C. Depression.
   D. Acceptance.

ACTIVITY 3 – TRUE/FALSE

In the space provided, write T if you think the statement is true or F if you think the statement is false.

1. _____ Everyone believes in life after death.

2. _____ Many people fear death because they are afraid of the unknown.

3. _____ The first stage of grief is bargaining.

4. _____ We all go through the stages of grief in an orderly progression.

5. _____ Bereavement is a period of grief someone goes through after a loved one dies.

6. _____ End of life care is the same as palliative care.

7. _____ Medicare covers hospice care for people who will die within 6 months.

8. _____ By forcing them to face reality, you help a dying resident reach acceptance.

9. _____ Reflection is a communication technique that may help a resident to talk about their feelings.

10. _____ The statement "I want to see my grandson graduate college," is an example of denial.

11. _____ If a dying resident seems unhappy with everything you do, they may be in the stage of anger.

12. _____ Family members of a dying resident always lose control of their emotions.

13. _____ It's OK to gossip about a resident after they have passed away.

14. _____ Just before death, a resident's eyes may stare blankly into space, with no eye movement.

15. _____ A resident's dentures should be discarded after death.

ACTIVITY 4 – SITUATION/RESPONSE

Read each situation. Write the letter of the appropriate response in the space provided.

Situation	Response
1. _____ Mrs. Littleton's roommate is very close to death. Mrs. Littleton seems agitated and upset, but doesn't seem willing to talk about her feelings.	A. Let the charge nurse know what you've observed. She may choose to talk with the resident's daughter about the stages of grief. The resident seems to be in denial.
2. _____ Mrs. Jackson is visiting her mother, who has been lingering close to death for a week. Mrs. Jackson has lost control of her emotions and is crying uncontrollably.	B. Respect her beliefs about reincarnation. Listen attentively when she talks, but don't force a discussion about your viewpoint.
3. _____ Mr. Montgomery has recently been told his lung cancer has spread to his liver and stomach. He has never seemed more cheerful. When his daughter tries to talk to him about signing an advance directive, he becomes angry and changes the subject.	C. Share your feelings with a trusted co-worker or friend. Remember that this is an awkward and painful time for the family. They may not ever thank you for all you have done for their loved one. You may have to comfort yourself by remembering the nice times you shared with the resident.
4. _____ Mrs. Spencer tells you that in a previous life she was a spiritual healer for a tribe of ancient Indians. You think this is ridiculous.	D. Give her an opportunity to open up about her feelings. Say something like, "You and your roommate have been such good friends; you must be very sad right now." If she doesn't want to talk, don't try to make her do so.
5. _____ One of your favorite residents is very close to death. You have been an important person in her life for over 2 years, but the family is ignoring you during these final hours. Your feelings are hurt.	E. Guide her to a private or secluded area. Offer her a tissue. Pay attention to her non-verbal communication. If she seems to want privacy, leave her alone. If she wants you to stay, begin a conversation with a statement like, "This must be very difficult for you."

ACTIVITY 5 – QUESTIONS TO CONSIDER

1. Do you have any fears about death? What helps you manage these fears?

4. What are some ways you can assist the dying resident's family during the process of dying?

2. Have you had anyone close to you die? What did you feel when you learned about their death?

5. List some ways you can assist residents in coping with the death of another resident. What may be their major concerns?

3. What religious or other rituals were a part of your saying goodbye to your loved one? How did these rituals help?

6. How will you deal with residents dying? List ways you can cope.

PULLING IT ALL TOGETHER

ACTIVITY 1 – TRUE/FALSE

In the space provided, write T if you think the statement is true or F if you think the statement is false.

1. _____ You treat residents as individuals when you give care based on their preferences.

2. _____ "Prioritizing" means you should do the most difficult tasks last.

3. _____ The charge nurse can help you learn how to organize your time.

4. _____ You are mindful when you balance the skill and the art of caregiving.

5. _____ A primary responsibility of the night shift is to prepare paperwork for the next day.

6. _____ You should never do a task that is normally done on another shift.

7. _____ You typically give care to "easy" residents after first caring for ill residents.

8 _____ Time management is a critical skill for a nurse assistant.

9. _____ Sticking to a schedule is one of your primary responsibilities.

10. _____ Making rounds before you begin specific tasks is important.

ACTIVITY 2 – MULTIPLE CHOICE

Circle the letter next to the best answer.

1. If you want to get along with residents and co-workers, you should always be:
   A. Content.
   B. Confusing.
   C. Considerate.
   D. Conservative.

2. How can you be a mindful caregiver?
   A. Consider the resident's preferences.
   B. Keep your residents on a consistent schedule.
   C. If a resident can't do a task quickly, do it for them.
   D. Never let a resident wear a dress twice in one week.

3. Using time management skills can help you avoid:
   A. Feeling unhappy.
   B. Feeling nauseous.
   C. Feeling disorganized.
   D. Feeling unappreciated.

4. How should you prioritize tasks?
   A. By the tasks that take the least time.
   B. By the tasks that need to be done soonest.
   C. By the tasks left over from the previous shift.
   D. By the order in which your co-worker does them.

5. Why is it critical to learn time management skills?
   A. So you never have to come in on your day off.
   B. So you have time to meet each resident's needs.
   C. So that you can leave work early when you want.
   D. So you have a chance to be employee of the month.

Decide which resident you should care for first and place a 1 by their name, a 2 by the resident you would assist next, and a 3 by the name of the resident you would assist last.

Case Study A

It is 8 a.m. and 3 residents need your attention all at once:

1. _____ Mrs. Siegelman is going to the hospital for an MRI at 9:30 a.m. She needs assistance bathing and dressing.

2. _____ Mr. Riley is anxious to take part in an activity later this morning. He needs your assistance to change clothes and has already asked for your help twice.

3. _____ Mrs. Byrne is confined to bed and has mild dementia. She hasn't eaten her breakfast yet because she needs assistance with feeding.

Case Study B

It is 5:45 p.m. and the evening is not going smoothly:

1. _____ Mr. Sessions is going to dinner with his daughter at 6 p.m. He was ready to go when he had an accident in his pants.

2. _____ Mrs. Miller was admitted today. Dinner is already being served in the dining room, and she won't come out of her room.

3. _____ Mr. Dupree has just returned from a visit with his grandchildren and has vomited on himself and the hallway floor.

Case Study C

It is 6 a.m. and your shift is going to be busy up until the end:

1. _____ Mrs. Harrison began coughing up blood during the night. Her son will arrive shortly to take her to the hospital for tests. She needs assistance dressing.

2. _____ Mrs. Daugherty has been up all night and seems agitated. She is at the desk asking for coffee.

3. _____ Mr. Lucas has moderate dementia. He has taken all his pajamas off and is standing in the doorway of the tub room.

ACTIVITY 4 – MATCHING

Read the descriptions of residents you've been assigned to care for on your shift. You need information from the charge nurse before you begin providing care. In the space provided, write the letter of the question that pertains to that resident.

Resident	Question for the Charge Nurse
1. ____ You will care for Mrs. Dahlgren this evening. At report you learned she only ate 50% of her breakfast and didn't touch her lunch.	A. Is this resident able to ambulate with assistance?
2. ____ You learned at report that Mr. Simmons was up all night. He has orders to go to physical therapy in the morning and you usually assist him with walking 2 times each day.	B. Should this resident receive the usual amount of exercise today?
3. ____ Mrs. Mattson had hip replacement surgery. She has been going to physical therapy once a day and sitting up in a chair for 2 hours each day. You are supposed to assist her with walking, but yesterday she refused to walk.	C. Is it o.k. for this resident to eat?
4. ____ Mrs. Jackson has complained of a stomach ache all day. She states that she is hungry now and would like to eat dinner.	D. Should I offer this resident a snack before dinner?
5. ____ Mr. Rutledge is having surgery in the morning. He is NPO p MN.	E. Is there anything I should do for this resident this evening?

ACTIVITY 5 – PRIORITIZING TASKS

For each situation below, decide the order in which tasks should be completed. Write a 1 beside the task you would do first, a 2 beside the task you would do next, and a 3 by the task you would do last. Any task you put off to the last may have to be done by the next shift.

Task List A

It is 6 a.m. and you must complete the following tasks:

1. _____ Mrs. Neilsen is having minor surgery today. She will be picked up at 7 a.m. You have to assist her with bathing and dressing.

2. _____ You must complete the 24-hour intake and output records for all your residents.

3. _____ Three of your residents rise around 6 a.m. and like to receive a.m. care right away.

Task List B

It is 1 p.m. and you must complete the following tasks:

1. _____ Give supplements to 3 residents and monitor their intake.

2. _____ Assist 2 residents with walking.

3. _____ Transfer vital signs and input/output information from your note pad to the appropriate charts.

Task List C

It is 10:30 p.m. and you must complete the following tasks:

1. _____ Offer a snack and beverage to 3 residents who are NPO p MN.

2. _____ Change the linens on an empty bed after a pitcher of water was accidentally spilled on them.

3. _____ Sit with a resident whose son just passed away suddenly.

ACTIVITY 6 – RESPONSIBILITY REVIEW

1. Give an example of a shift-related responsibility for the 7 a.m. to 3:30 p.m. shift.

2. Give an example of a shift-related responsibility for the 3 p.m. to 11:30 p.m. shift.

3. Give an example of a shift-related responsibility for the 11 p.m. to 7:30 a.m. shift.

ACTIVITY 7 — QUESTION & ANSWER

Using your own words, write an answer to each question.

1. What must you do before you can put a plan in place for providing care?

2. What does it mean to prioritize?

3. How well do you manage your time and yourself? Consider your personal and professional responsibilities, then develop a plan and write it below.

Chapter

PROMOTING YOUR OWN HEALTH

In the space provided, write the letter of the correct definition.

Term	Definition
1. _____ Aerobic	A. A mental state; the way life is viewed
2. _____ Anaerobic	B. Exercise that does not increase the supply of oxygen to the body tissue
3. _____ Attitude	C. A way of living
4. _____ Health promotion	D. Process of working to achieve a state of health and well-being
5. _____ Healthy lifestyle	E. Steady exercise that increases the heart rate and the amount of oxygen delivered to body tissue

ACTIVITY 2 – CONTENT REVIEW

List 8 lifestyle factors that can influence your health. Refer to the textbook if necessary. Hint: one lifestyle factor is to wear your seatbelt.

1. _____

2. _____

3. _____

4. _____

5. _____

6. _____

7. _____

8. _____

List 5 ways to keep a positive attitude. Refer to the textbook if necessary. Hint: one way is to "see the glass half full, not half empty."

9. _____

10. _____

11. _____

12. _____

13. _____

ACTIVITY 3 – MULTIPLE CHOICE

Circle the letter beside the best answer.

1. Complete the following sentence. Good health depends on:
   A. Eating liver and spinach everyday.
   B. Drinking 8 oz of orange juice everyday.
   C. Staying very thin and avoiding carbohydrates.
   D. Good nutrition, regular exercise, and a positive attitude.

2. According to the food pyramid, which food group has the most recommended servings?
   A. Dairy
   B. Fruits
   C. Grains
   D. Vegetables

3. Women should limit their alcohol consumption to no more than:
   A. 1 drink per day
   B. 2 drinks per day
   C. 1 drink per week
   D. 2 drinks per week

4. What does the word "aerobic" mean?
   A. Healthy.
   B. With oxygen.
   C. Without oxygen.
   D. Outdoor activity.

5. When you exercise regularly, you help maintain joint flexibility and mobility. What kinds of problems can flexibility and mobility prevent?
   A. Poor vision.
   B. Skin cancer.
   C. Contractures.
   D. Forgetfulness.

ACTIVITY 4 – CONTENT REVIEW

In the left hand column, list the 5 food groups from the USDA food pyramid. In the right hand column, list the number of daily servings suggested for that category. Use your textbook if necessary.

Food Group   Servings

1a. _____   1b. _____

2a. _____   2b. _____

3a. _____   3b. _____

4a. _____   4b. _____

5a. _____   5b. _____

ACTIVITY 5 – HABITS TO CONSIDER

For 2 days, keep a journal and write down everything that you eat, the exercise you get, and special activities that you enjoy. After 2 days, make lists of the following:

1. What I can do to exercise:

_____

_____

_____

2. How I can improve what I eat:

_____

_____

_____

3. Nice things I can do for myself:

_____

_____

_____

ACTIVITY 6 – CRITICAL THINKING

List some reasons why you think some people do not live a healthy lifestyle. For each of the reasons you list, describe a way to change. Note the example provided.

No time to exercise.

Take a walk at lunchtime instead of eating dessert.

_____

_____

_____

_____

_____

_____

_____

_____

In your own words, describe good nutrition.

_____

_____

_____

_____

_____

Describe the benefits of exercise.

_____

_____

_____

_____

_____

Chapter 27

HOW TO BE A SUCCESSFUL EMPLOYEE

ACTIVITY 1 – SPELL IT OUT

Using the terms and clues provided complete the spelling of each word.

Aggressive   Assertive   Competency   Initiative

1. Abilities that are legally required or shown to be adequate: _____ M _____ N _____

2. Behavior in which you speak up for yourself without hurting others: _____ S _____ E

3. Attempting to take the first step to settle an issue: _____ I _____ V __

4. Behavior that is hurtful to others and may make them angry: _____ R ___ S _____

ACTIVITY 2 – TRUE/FALSE

Read each statement. In the space provided, write T if the statement is true or F if the statement is false.

1. _____ Once a nurse assistant has passed the state exam, they know everything they need to do their job.

2. _____ Most nurse assistants who do well in training also do well on the state exam.

3. _____ No matter who you are or how much you know, you always can learn something new.

4. _____ For most people, starting a new job isn't stressful.

5. _____ For a nurse assistant, the chain of command begins with the director of food services.

6. _____ When you act assertively, you always get what you want.

7. _____ When you act aggressively, people will respect you.

8. _____ Feedback from residents and co-workers can help you improve your work.

ACTIVITY 3 – CONTENT REVIEW

Complete each list, referring to your textbook as needed.

Part A

List 5 steps you can take to keep yourself motivated on the job. Hint: one step is to stay healthy.

1. _____

2. _____

3. _____

4. _____

5. _____

Part B

List 5 habits that can make your job unpleasant. Hint: one habit is gossiping about residents or staff.

1. _____

2. _____

3. _____

4. _____

5. _____

ACTIVITY 4 – YES OR NO

Read over the following suggestions for preparing for the state exam. If it is an effective strategy, write YES in the space provided. If it is a not an effective strategy, write NO.

1. _____ Get a good night's sleep before the exam.

2. _____ Have all the necessary documents with you.

3. _____ Eat a well-balanced meal before the exam.

4. _____ Practice skills with a friend or co-worker.

5. _____ Have several glasses of wine to relax you before the exam.

6. _____ Obtain a sample test and complete it.

7. _____ Review the text and what you learned during training.

8. _____ Cross your fingers and hope for the best.

ACTIVITY 5 – MULTIPLE CHOICE

Circle the letter beside the best answer.

1. How can you create a good first impression with a potential employer?
   A. Take a box of candy as a gesture of friendship.
   B. Take your best friend with you when you interview.
   C. Fill out the employment application neatly and accurately.
   D. Tell them what you didn't like about your previous supervisors.

2. Once you begin working as a nurse assistant, you can expect to:
   A. Know everything you need to know.
   B. Receive an orientation to the new job.
   C. Feel completely comfortable in your new role.
   D. Feel completely at ease with residents and families the first day.

3. How can you stay motivated on the job?
   A. Do no more than what the job requires.
   B. Take advantage of all opportunities to learn.
   C. Ignore the people and co-workers you don't like.
   D. Find a resident who will listen to your complaints.

4. Following the chain of command, what is your first step in resolving a grievance or concern about your work?
   A. Talking to the housekeeper.
   B. Talking to the charge nurse.
   C. Talking to the social worker.
   D. Talking to the administrator.

5. What is the best way to know if you're doing a good job?
   A. Assume that people will tell you if you make a mistake.
   B. Do your job the way other nurse assistants do theirs.
   C. Ask residents, families, and co-workers for feedback.
   D. Ask others to complete a survey about your performance.

ACTIVITY 6 –MATCHING

Read each statement or action. In the space provided, write AG if the statement or action is aggressive, AS if it is assertive, or P if it is passive.

AGGRESSIVE   ASSERTIVE   PASSIVE

You work the evening shift and you've completed all the normal tasks before taking your dinner break. You've helped all of your residents get ready for bed, passed around snacks and supplements, and completed your paperwork. Your co-worker is running behind schedule. You've seen her chatting on the phone and watched her flip through a magazine in the break room. Now she has asked if you will help her complete her tasks so the 2 of you can go to dinner together. You are hungry and you resent the fact that she's wasted her time while you made good use of yours.

1. _____ You sigh and shrug your shoulders, put your dinner away, and ask her what needs to be done.

2. _____ You explain that you've completed your work and that you're going to take your break now.

3. _____ You shake your finger in her face as you tell her that you've watched her waste time all evening and that it's not your responsibility to help her do her job.

Mrs. Lane's daughter discovers that one of her mother's nicest dresses has a rip in it. Mrs. Lane, who is confused, tells the daughter you caused the tear. You have no idea how or when the dress was torn.

4. _____ You say, "I have no idea when or how it was torn, but I'm sorry it happened to such a pretty dress. Would you like to talk to the charge nurse about this?"

5. _____ You say, "Your mother doesn't have a clue what's going on around her, so how can you accuse me of tearing the dress? If you don't like the way I do my job, you should speak to the charge nurse."

6. _____ You say, "It was probably my fault. I'm really sorry."

ACTIVITY 7 – QUESTIONS TO CONSIDER

Using your own words, answer the following questions.

As a result of taking this course, what new information did you learn about residents in nursing facilities?

_____

_____

_____

What new information did you learn about yourself?

_____

_____

What can you do if you find yourself unhappy in your job?

_____

_____

What are some ways you can continue to learn on the job?

_____

_____

Practice Exam

Circle the letter beside the best answer.

1. Which of these services is usually provided in a long term care facility?
   A. Home health care.
   B. Radiation therapy.
   C. Rehabilitative care.
   D. Surgery.

2. What is an example of mindful caregiving?
   A. Being on time for work.
   B. Encouraging residents to wear clothing you like.
   C. Observing changes in a resident's mood or routine.
   D. Requiring a resident to stick with the facility's schedule.

3. What is an effective way to get to know a resident?
   A. Discuss the resident with housekeeping staff.
   B. Read the resident's mail and personal papers.
   C. Ask the resident about their needs and preferences.
   D. Check with the resident's roommate for information.

4. Which of these is an example of negligence?
   A. Teasing a resident in an unkind manner.
   B. Threatening a resident with physical harm.
   C. Locking a resident in their room against their will.
   D. Not taking a resident to the bathroom when they ask.

5. Which of these statements about our perceptions is true?
   A. Our perceptions about residents are always accurate.
   B. We should always believe that what we perceive is true, regardless of whether it may be right or wrong.
   C. Our perceptions influence how we behave toward others.
   D. Single-minded perceptions of residents help us get to know them better.

6. How can you make a new resident feel that they belong?
   A. Call them by the nickname "honey."
   B. Encourage them to participate in activities.
   C. Ask if you can borrow some of their jewelry.
   D. Leave them alone to adjust to the facility on their own.

7. Which of the following symptoms is typical of mid-stage dementia?
   A. Loss of appetite.
   B. Tendency to feel cold most of the time.
   C. Great difficulty making decisions.
   D. Improved recent memory.

8. Which of these nonverbal behaviors helps develop a positive relationship with a resident?
   A. Smiling warmly.
   B. Always keeping your facial expressions neutral.
   C. Looking over the resident's shoulder when you speak to them.
   D. Folding your arms across your chest.

9. What is the purpose of a living will?
   A. To settle property and financial issues when a person dies.
   B. To help family members decide how they want their loved one cared for.
   C. To keep family members away from a dying resident.
   D. To guide decisions about a person's care if they become incapacitated.

10. You're involved in an argument with a co-worker. In order to resolve the conflict, you should:
    A. Tell the co-worker what's wrong with their point of view.
    B. Bring up past conflicts you've had with the co-worker.
    C. Take time to understand the other person's point of view.
    D. Calm things down by joking about their point of view.

11. A resident's care plan is used as a tool to:
    A. Determine whether the resident qualifies for Medicaid payments.
    B. Invite family members to facility parties.
    C. Plan for new building improvements.
    D. Coordinate all treatments and services for the resident.

12. How residents perceive and respond to pain is influenced by:
    A. Their nutritional status.
    B. Sunlight.
    C. The clothing they are wearing at the time.
    D. Their cultural or religious background and beliefs.

13. Whenever you prepare to do a task, you should ask yourself a number of questions, including which of the following?
    A. Is this task in my job description?
    B. Did I get the resident's permission to do the task?
    C. Should I call the resident's family to check whether they want me to do this task?
    D. Will the charge nurse respect me more for doing this task?

14. You can help to break the chain of infection at each link by:
    A. Sterilizing all bed linen every morning.
    B. Disinfecting all surfaces.
    C. Wearing a gown and protective eyewear at all times.
    D. Washing your hands before and after every contact with a resident.

15. When a family member is angry or critical, you should:
    A. Take their comments personally.
    B. Explain that the facility is understaffed and there's nothing anyone can do.
    C. Be supportive and report the situation to the charge nurse.
    D. Pretend you agree with them that the facility is not doing a good job.

16. Your role in helping maintain a resident's nutrition includes:
    A. Planning meals for the week.
    B. Helping food service staff prepare meals.
    C. Insisting that residents eat everything on their plate.
    D. Serving meals while hot foods are still hot and cold foods are cold.

17. To make sure a resident is safe during a bath, you should:
    A. Close the tub room door.
    B. Undress the resident in the tub room.
    C. Check the water temperature.
    D. Remove all your jewelry.

18. As a nurse assistant, you typically learn about a resident's symptoms by:
    A. Interviewing the resident's roommate.
    B. Talking to the resident.
    C. Observing the resident while they sleep.
    D. Taking the resident's vital signs.

19. Which of the following occurs because of nervous system changes as we age?
    A. Slowing of respirations.
    B. Slowing of heartbeat.
    C. Decreased insulin production.
    D. Decreased short-term memory.

20. The Heimlich maneuver is used with a resident who is:
    A. Vomiting.
    B. Having a seizure.
    C. Choking.
    D. Feeling nauseous.

21. How can you help a resident be independent?
    A. Select their clothing for them each day.
    B. Encourage the resident to do what they can.
    C. Insist on helping them with bathing.
    D. Leave them alone to take care of themselves.

22. The Resident's Bill of Rights includes:
    A. The right to have a private room.
    B. The right to be happy all the time.
    C. The right to privacy and confidentiality.
    D. The right to receive all services free of charge.

23. The nurse asks you to give ROM exercise to a resident who is confined to bed. According to her care plan, there are no restrictions. What does "no restrictions" mean?
    A. You should work their joints and muscles very hard.
    B. Provide ROM exercise as often as possible on each shift.
    C. The resident should be able to all of the exercises alone.
    D. You may move each joint through its full available range.

24. Mr. Nathanson is experiencing a seizure and you have called for help. What else should you do for him?
    A. Pour water into his mouth.
    B. Help him to the floor to prevent a fall.
    C. Put a toothbrush or something firm between his teeth for him to bite on.
    D. Ask other residents to help you hold him down firmly.

25. When you maintain the resident's privacy during all aspects of personal care, which theme of care are you paying attention to?
    A. Respect.
    B. Safety.
    C. Communication.
    D. Infection control.

26. Using good body mechanics will help you:
    A. Get all your work done before your shift ends.
    B. Lose weight.
    C. Avoid injuries.
    D. Develop stronger muscles.

27. You should check a resident's vital signs:
    A. Only on the first day of each month.
    B. Whenever a change occurs that might signal an illness.
    C. Everyday at the beginning of your shift.
    D. Only when the charge nurse tells you to.

28. If a resident starts to feel dizzy as you help them stand up from their bed to get to their walker, you should:
    A. Move them quickly to the walker before they have a chance to fall.
    B. Help them to lie down in bed and call for the charge nurse.
    C. Keep them standing for a minute until the dizziness passes.
    D. Have them sit on the edge of the bed while you go to talk to the charge nurse.

29. Your role in the care plan meeting includes:
    A. Sharing information about the resident.
    B. Serving coffee and doughnuts to the interdisciplinary team.
    C. Deciding which doctors and nurses should attend.
    D. Diagnosing the resident's medical condition.

30. When you position a resident on their side, their legs should normally be positioned:
    A. With a pillow between them.
    B. However the charge nurse tells you.
    C. With both legs straight and slightly apart.
    D. With one leg straight and one leg slightly bent.

31. When you provide personal care, it is important to:
    A. Have all morning care done before 8 a.m.
    B. Never give care that has not been clearly requested by the family.
    C. Keep on schedule, even if you have to rush slow residents.
    D. Encourage the resident to do all that they can for themselves.

32. How can you help a family get over their guilt when a resident is admitted into a long-term care facility?
    A. Encourage them to question their decision to admit their family member.
    B. Give their family member the best care you can.
    C. Tell them they are in charge of bathing and dressing their family member whenever they visit.
    D. Just nod and smile whenever they make suggestions about their loved one's care.

33. What is a common cause of a decubitus ulcer?
    A. Uncomfortable clothing.
    B. Dirty pajamas.
    C. Pressure on the skin.
    D. Stress caused by family arguments.

34. What is a benefit of observing residents carefully while providing personal care?
    A. It frees you from having to observe residents at other times.
    B. You have the opportunity to talk with residents about family members.
    C. You may note both physical and psychological changes in residents.
    D. You can decide whether or not to give residents their medications, depending on how they feel.

35. Why is it important reason to make a neat, wrinkle free bed?
    A. Wrinkles give germs places to grow.
    B. It is more difficult to launder sheets that become very wrinkled.
    C. Wrinkled sheets can cause skin irritation and breakdown.
    D. Old-fashioned charge nurses think neat beds look better.

36. The signs and symptoms of dehydration may include:
    A. Blurred vision.
    B. Rosy pink skin color.
    C. Decreased urine output.
    D. Elevated blood pressure.

37. Why is it important to be familiar with a resident's elimination pattern?
    A. So that you never have to clean up an accident.
    B. So that you can recognize and report any changes.
    C. To keep the family informed at every visit.
    D. Because you discuss every resident's elimination at the end of your shift.

38. Why is it good practice to use a guard belt when transferring a resident?
    A. You never need other helpers.
    B. It helps to support the resident's body during the transfer.
    C. It keeps the resident's clothing in place during the transfer.
    D. It makes the transfer go twice as fast.

39. You are a new nurse assistant at your facility. How might you learn that a certain resident has frequent incontinence?
    A. By checking the resident's medical record.
    B. By interviewing all family members that come to visit the resident.
    C. By sneaking into the resident's room at lunch to check the sheets for dampness.
    D. By asking the laundry to check the resident's clothing for urine stains.

40. When you give ROM exercises, it is important to:
    A. Wear gloves and a gown.
    B. Exercise the resident at least until they begin to sweat.
    C. Follow the therapist's written plan.
    D. Move each joint just to the point where it begins to be painful.

41. What is an ICF/MR?
    A. A nursing facility that cares for residents who are mentally retarded.
    B. A specialized facility that provides care for an elderly disabled person.
    C. A congregate care facility for elderly residents with diabetes.
    D. A facility that provides a home-like environment for people in wheelchairs.

42. A resident's daughter complains to you that you ask her mother to bathe herself. How should you answer the daughter?
    A. You have a lot of people to care for and don't have time for everyone.
    B. You suggest the daughter care for the mother herself.
    C. You ask the daughter file a formal complaint.
    D. You explain you are helping her mother maintain her independence.

43. You are communicating assertively when you:
    A. Feel guilty after saying you cannot volunteer for an extra shift.
    B. Share your complaints with residents.
    C. Speak up for yourself without hurting others.
    D. Say what you think other people will want to hear.

44. To prevent a stage one pressure ulcer from getting worse, you should:
    A. Frequently give the resident ice chips to suck on.
    B. Give the resident three vitamin pills daily.
    C. Follow the charge nurse's instructions.
    D. Cover the area with a warm, moist cloth at all times.

45. Why is it important to wear gloves when you provide mouth care?
    A. So you won't have to wash your hands.
    B. The resident may have a cold.
    C. In case the resident's gums bleed.
    D. In case you get toothpaste on your hands.

46. When a resident with an infection is on contact precautions, you should:
    A. Never allow any visitors under any circumstances.
    B. Request that the charge nurse provide all care.
    C. Wear gloves when providing care.
    D. Install a special air ventilation system.

47. How can you help a resident manage their pain?
    A. Make the lights in their room as bright as possible.
    B. Report any signs or symptoms of pain to the charge nurse.
    C. Offer them plenty of snacks and beverages between meals.
    D. Turn the television up loud.

48. Which of the following techniques is helpful when you are dealing with an agitated resident?
    A. Yelling.
    B. Distraction.
    C. Reality orientation.
    D. Clapping your hands and stomping your foot.

49. Which of the following is a developmentally disabled person?
    A. A person who lost use of their legs after a car accident.
    B. An elderly person who has developed Alzheimer's disease.
    C. A person with a chronic, severe condition that developed in childhood.
    D. A frail elderly person who needs assistance with bathing and dressing.

50. You can help a dying resident cope with their feelings by:
    A. Discouraging them from talking about painful topics.
    B. Using techniques of reality orientation.
    C. Explaining your own views about death.
    D. Listening to what they have to say.

51. After you make rounds, you prioritize your tasks based on:
    A. Which tasks require the most supplies.
    B. Which tasks can be completed most quickly.
    C. What tasks you'll have to leave for the next shift.
    D. Which residents require the most assistance.

52. How can you demonstrate your desire to be a good employee?
    A. Be late to work no more than once a week.
    B. Record care activities in the resident's medical record even before you have done them.
    C. Cooperate with other team members.
    D. Offer to share your lunch with other nurse assistants.

53. You should limit your daily intake of total fat to:
    A. 30% or less of your total calories.
    B. 40% or less of your total calories.
    C. 50% or less of your total calories.
    D. 60% or less of your total calories.

54. Which of these tasks is performed by nursing staff?
   A. Prescribing medications.
   B. Giving medications.
   C. Planning menus for the whole facility.
   D. Repairing medical equipment.

55. What is "mindful caregiving?"
   A. Wearing comfortable shoes and clothing to work.
   B. Storing soiled equipment and supplies in the clean supply room.
   C. Paying attention to details and being open, observant, and flexible.
   D. Sharing your opinions about a resident's care with their family members.

56. To become or stay physically fit you should:
   A. Exercise only if your doctor says you need to.
   B. Exercise 1 minute per pound per day that you are overweight.
   C. Exercise at least 30 minutes 3 or 4 times a week.
   D. Exercise a minimum of an hour every day.

57. Inservice education is important because:
   A. It prepares you for the nurse assistant exam that you have to take every year.
   B. You get paid more for every hour of inservice you take.
   C. The nurse assistants with the most hours of inservice get to pick their shifts.
   D. It gives you an opportunity to grow, change, and improve.

58. Aging changes happen to everyone. Which of these changes is also a normal part of aging?
   A. The need to be fed.
   B. An inability to walk.
   C. Thinning of the skin.
   D. The loss of one's teeth.

59. Walkers, canes, and crutches are examples of which type of device?
   A. Orthotic.
   B. Assistive.
   C. Listening.
   D. Prosthetic.

60. When caring for a resident you must consider:
   A. Your own schedule.
   B. Your own preferences.
   C. The resident's preferences.
   D. The housekeeping schedule.

Answer Sheet

1. _____
2. _____
3. _____
4. _____
5. _____
6. _____
7. _____
8. _____
9. _____
10. _____
11. _____
12. _____
13. _____
14. _____
15. _____
16. _____
17. _____
18. _____
19. _____
20. _____
21. _____
22. _____
23. _____
24. _____
25. _____
26. _____
27. _____
28. _____
29. _____
30. _____

31. _____
32. _____
33. _____
34. _____
35. _____
36. _____
37. _____
38. _____
39. _____
40. _____
41. _____
42. _____
43. _____
44. _____
45. _____
46. _____
47. _____
48. _____
49. _____
50. _____
51. _____
52. _____
53. _____
54. _____
55. _____
56. _____
57. _____
58. _____
59. _____
60. _____

SKILLS CHECKLISTS

PROCEDURE 9-1 – HANDWASHING

Note: *Check the sink, soap dispenser, and towel dispenser before beginning. Ask yourself: "Will I contaminate my hands touching these items after I wash my hands?" If your answer is yes, prepare these before you begin.*

1. ____ Remove your watch and roll up your sleeves. **Note:** *You may not want to wear jewelry so you don't have to constantly remove it for handwashing. If you do not remove your watch and rings, be sure to wash, rinse, and dry under them.*
2. ____ Turn on the water to a comfortable temperature. Wet your hands and wrists.
3. ____ Apply soap to your hands.
4. ____ Rub your hands together in a circular motion with friction for 10-15 seconds. Lace your fingers together to wash in between them). Clean under your fingernails: Use a nail brush or orange stick, or rub your nails briskly in your palm to clean them. **Note:** *Because acrylic or silk-wrap (artificial) nails are difficult to clean under and may harbor bacteria, they should not be worn.*
5. ____ Rinse your hands with warm water, keeping them downward, allowing the water to run from the wrist to the fingers.
6. ____ Get paper towels from the dispenser. **Note:** *If you have to touch the dispenser to remove the towel, you must have the towel ready before you start so you do not contaminate your hands.*
7. ____ Dry your hands with paper towels. Start at the top of the fingers and work downward toward the wrists.
8. ____ Turn off the faucets with a paper towel.
9. ____ Discard paper towels in appropriate receptacle.

PROCEDURE 11-1 – COLLECTING A SPUTUM SPECIMEN

Note: *Make sure a resident who chews tobacco has not done so before you collect the specimen. If the resident has just eaten, ask them to rinse out their mouth. Try to collect the specimen in the morning. Often large amounts of sputum are coughed up first thing in the morning.*

1. ____ Give the resident the sputum collection container or hold it yourself. Take care not to touch its inside surface, or lining.
2. ____ Ask the resident to take deep breaths and cough deeply from the chest. They may need to cough several times to get enough sputum for the sample. Ask them to try not to spit only saliva into the container.
3. ____ Place the lid securely on the specimen bottle. Label it with the resident's name, room number, and the date and time of the collection. Place the specimen in a biohazardous bag.
4. ____ Report the color, amount, and consistency of the specimen to the charge nurse.

PROCEDURE 11-2 – APPLICATION OF SUPPORT HOSE AND ELASTIC STOCKINGS

1. ____ Wash, dry, and inspect the resident's legs and feet and between the toes.
2. ____ Put a small amount of powder on the resident's feet to help the stocking go on more easily.
3. ____ Before putting stockings on, turn each stocking inside out except for the toe.
4. ____ Securely put the toe in place and slide the stocking up over the heel. Be sure the heel is positioned properly in the stocking, and then carefully pull the stocking up and over the calf. Make sure there are no wrinkles in the stockings. Wrinkles or twists can cause pressure and decrease circulation. **Note:** *Remember that the resident's skin may be thin and fragile and can tear easily.*
5. ____ Put the other stocking on the other leg in the same manner.

PROCEDURE 11-3 – GIVING AN ENEMA

1. _____ Put on gloves.
2. _____ Place disposable protective pad under the resident's buttocks. Place a second protective pad at the end of the bed to place under and over bedpan when resident is finished.
3. _____ Position the resident on their left side, helping them turn if necessary. Make sure their hips are near the edge of the bed on the side where you're working.
4. _____ Hold the rectal tube over the bedpan. Open the clamp on the tubing and let the solution run through into the bedpan until it flows smoothly, so that no air is left in the tubing to cause discomfort for the resident. Close the clamp.
5. _____ Turn back the bath blanket so that the resident's hips are exposed but the rest of the body is covered. Hold the lubricated rectal tube about 5 inches from the tip. Gently put it into the rectum to the red line on the tube.
6. _____ Raise the container about 15 inches above the resident's hips. Never hold the container any higher.
7. _____ Open the clamp and let the solution run in slowly. If the resident complains of cramps, tell them to breathe deeply through their mouth, as you clamp the tubing for a minute or so. You may also lower the irrigating bag.
8. _____ When all the solution has run in, close the clamp.
9. _____ Remove the rectal tube. Place the tubing in a plastic trash bag.
10. _____ Turn the resident on their back and slip the bedpan under them. Ask the resident to try to hold the solution as long as possible. Raise the head of the bed. Ensure that the call button and toilet paper are within reach.
11. _____ Give the resident privacy, but do not leave them for a long period of time. Check on the resident after 5 minutes.
12. _____ When the resident feels they are done, put on gloves, and assist with wiping if necessary. Remove the bedpan and place it on a protective pad. Remove your gloves, and help the resident into a comfortable position. Put on gloves and remove the covered bedpan.

PROCEDURE 11-4 – APPLYING A DISPOSABLE INCONTINENCE BRIEF

1. _____ Place an incontinence pad on the bed to protect clean linen.
2. _____ Help the resident onto their back.
3. _____ Put on gloves.
4. _____ Help remove garments below the waist.
5. _____ Discard the soiled incontinence brief in the plastic trash bag.
6. _____ Remove and dispose of your soiled gloves.
7. _____ Put on new gloves.
8. _____ With the resident on their side, give perineal care, including cleaning the rectal area.
9. _____ Remove and dispose of your soiled gloves.
10. _____ Put on new gloves.
11. _____ Fan-fold one-half of the briefs under the resident's buttocks.
12. _____ Help the resident move onto their back. Unfold the side that was fan-folded, and open the adhesive tabs on both sides. Place the brief upward between the resident's legs, and join the tab from the back of the brief to the tab in the front of the brief.
13. _____ Put on the resident's underpants and clothing.

PROCEDURE 11-5 – EMPTYING A CATHETER DRAINAGE BAG

1. _____ Put on gloves.
2. _____ Place the paper towel on the floor underneath the drainage bag.
3. _____ Place the measuring container on the paper towel.
4. _____ The drainage bag has a closed clamp that allows the urine to flow from the bag. Open the clamp and drain all the urine into the container, making sure not to touch the clamp to the sides of the container.
5. _____ Close the clamp and secure it to the drainage bag immediately after it is completely drained.
6. _____ Note the amount of urine and discard the urine in the resident's toilet.
7. _____ Remove and discard your gloves, and wash your hands.
8. _____ Record the amount of urine on the intake and output record.

PROCEDURE 14-1 – TAKING AN ORAL TEMPERATURE

Note: *Check with the person to make sure they have not just eaten or drunk something hot or cold or smoked a cigarette in the last 10 minutes. These activities change the temperature of the mouth and give you a false reading. If they did, wait 5-10 minutes.*

1. _____ Shake the thermometer down to 95 F or to the lowest number, and then put on the plastic cover.
2. _____ Insert the bulb end of the thermometer under the resident's tongue, and ask them to close their lips around it. The resident may want to hold onto the end of the thermometer to keep it in place. The resident should not walk with the thermometer in their mouth.
3. _____ Wait at least 3 minutes. As you wait, you can take the person's pulse and respiratory rates. Remove the thermometer and the plastic cover. Read the temperature. **Note:** *If there is an excessive amount of mucus on the thermometer when you remove it, use a barrier such as gloves to remove the cover.*
4. _____ If you use an electronic thermometer, wait until it beeps.
5. _____ Record the result.

PROCEDURE 14-2 – TAKING A RECTAL TEMPERATURE

1. _____ Be sure to wear gloves.
2. _____ Shake down the thermometer to 95 F or lower.
3. _____ Position the resident on either side. Help the resident bend up the upper leg as far as possible.
4. _____ Put a plastic cover (if used) over the thermometer and lubricate it. Separate the person's buttocks with one hand while with the other you insert the bulb 1 inch into the rectum.
5. _____ Hold the thermometer in place 1 to 3 minutes, remove it, and wipe any excess lubricant from the rectum with a piece of tissue paper. Remove the cover, and read the thermometer.
6. _____ Record the result.

Note: *Always cover a resident while taking a rectal temperature. Never leave them during this time because they may roll off their side and be injured by the thermometer. Talk with the person while waiting for the temperature reading to take their mind off the procedure.*

PROCEDURE 14-3. – TAKING AN AXILLARY TEMPERATURE

1. _____ Shake down the thermometer to 95 F or lower.
2. _____ Loosen the resident's clothing to be able to reach the armpit. Dry the armpit.
3. _____ Place the thermometer in the resident's armpit. Have them place the arm down along their side.
4. _____ Wait 10 minutes. Remove the thermometer and read the temperature.
5. _____ Record the result.

PROCEDURE 14-4. – TAKING A RADIAL PULSE

1. _____ Place your second and third fingers gently over the radial artery (on the thumb side of the wrist) and note the rhythm of the pulse.
2. _____ Look at your watch, and when the second hand is on the 12, start counting the pulse for 1 minute. Count each beat you feel. Check for abnormalities in the rhythm.
3. _____ Record the result.

PROCEDURE 14-5. – TAKING A RESPIRATORY RATE

1. _____ Count the respiratory rate immediately after counting the pulse rate.
2. _____ Keep your fingers on the resident's radial pulse but without pressure. (Do this so the resident will breathe normally. Often residents hold their breath or breathe deeper if they know you are counting.) Watch the chest go up with inspiration and down with expiration.
3. _____ Count the respiratory rate for 1 minute.
4. _____ Record the result.

PROCEDURE 14-6. – TAKING A BLOOD PRESSURE

1. _____ Have the resident place their arm on the bed, bedside table, or arm of the chair, with their palm up and elbow at the same level as the heart. (If the arm is higher than the heart, the blood pressure can register too high. If the arm is lower than the heart, the blood pressure can register too low.)

2. _____ Expose the resident's arm by rolling the sleeve up to the shoulder, taking care that the sleeve is not too tight on the arm, which might increase the blood pressure. Wrap the blood pressure cuff evenly around the upper arm 1 inch above the elbow. Make sure the arm is not lying on the tubing and the tubing is not kinked. The tube that is attached to the bulb should be on the side closest to the resident's body. The tube to the sphygmomanometer gauge should be on the other side of the arm, away from the body. Be sure to use the correct size cuff for the resident. The wrong size cuff can give you an incorrect reading. The cuff should fit over the center of the resident's upper arm. It should not extend to the elbow or to under the resident's armpit.

3. _____ Close the valve in the air pump by turning it clockwise. The valve is the little metal knob on the bulb.

4. _____ Place the stethoscope earpieces in your ears.

5. _____ Locate the pulsation in the brachial artery by placing your second and third fingers over the area. When you find the pulse, place the diaphragm of the stethoscope firmly over the area and hold it in place with your left hand. Use your right hand if you are left-handed.

6. _____ With your right hand, pump air into the cuff by squeezing the bulb until the gauge measures 180–200. **Note.** *If you hear the pulse immediately after stopping pumping, begin again and pump the cuff so the gauge reads higher than 200 mm Hg (Hg=symbol for mercury). One way to avoid pumping the cuff too high is to feel the pulse at the brachial artery and pump the cuff slowly until you no longer feel the pulse, making sure to remember where you last felt the pulse and to add 30 mm Hg when beginning to take the blood pressure.*

7. _____ Slowly open the valve on the bulb and watch the cuff pressure decrease on the gauge.

8. _____ Listen for the first thumping sound and note the pressure reading; remember this number. This is the systolic pressure.

9. _____ Continue to listen for a distinct change in sound (muffled sounding) or the last sound and note the pressure reading. This is the diastolic pressure.

10. _____ Record the results.

PROCEDURE 14-7 – MAKING AN UNOCCUPIED BED

1. _____ Look for any belongings in the bed. Residents may fall asleep with personal belongings under their pillow or elsewhere in the bed.

2. _____ Lower the head of the bed and raise the whole bed to a comfortable position (usually about hip level).

3. _____ Remove the spread and any blankets, and fold them on the chair.

4. _____ Remove soiled linen, including the pillowcase. Loosen sheets from under the mattress and carefully roll them into a ball, keeping the soiled side inside the ball and away from your body. (This keeps the cleaner side close to you. Rolling linens prevents the spread of organisms from dirty linens.) Put the sheets in the laundry bag.

5. _____ Check the mattress for any soiling or wetness. Wash and dry it with paper towels if necessary. Change the mattress pad if it is soiled or scheduled for change.

6. _____ If you are using a fitted sheet (shaped to the mattress by elastic edging), follow these steps:
Starting at the top corner of the mattress, wrap the edge of the mattress with the corner of the sheet, then go to the bottom of bed on the same side and wrap that edge. Do not shake the linen while unfolding it. (Shaking the linen raises dust and organisms.) Go to the opposite corner at the top of the bed and wrap that edge, and then wrap the last edge over the last corner. The sheet should fit the mattress snugly.

7. _____ If you are using a draw sheet, follow these steps: place it in the center of the bed so it covers the middle part of the bed. Tuck in the draw sheet on both sides. A draw sheet is often used for residents needing help with moving and positioning, or to keep bottom sheets clean and dry.

8. If you are using a flat sheet follow these steps:

   a. Unfold the bottom sheet lengthwise down the bed's center. Do not shake the linen while unfolding it. (Shaking linen raises dust and organisms.) Put the hem seams toward the mattress This keeps rough edges from touching the person.

   b. Slide the sheet so that the hem is even with the foot of the mattress. Keep the fold in the exact center of the bed from head to foot. (You want the extra length of sheet at the top to tuck it under the mattress).

   c. Open the sheet from the fold so that the sheet covers the entire mattress and hangs evenly on both sides. Tuck the top hem in tightly under the mattress at the head of the bed by lifting the head of the mattress and sliding the sheet under the mattress. Make a mitered corner (also called a hospital corner):

      i. Face the side of the bed.

      ii. With one hand, pick up the top of the sheet hanging down the side of the bed, and lay it on top of the bed so that it looks like a triangle.

      iii. Tuck the remaining sheet under the mattress.

      iv. Drop the section of sheet from on top of the bed over the side of the bed, and tuck it in.

   d. Tuck the remaining sheet under the mattress neatly, starting from the mitered corner down to the foot of the mattress.

   e. If a draw sheet is used, open it up and place it in the center of the bed so it covers the middle part of the bed. Tuck in the draw sheet on each side. A draw sheet is often used for residents needing help with moving and positioning, or sometimes to keep bottom sheets clean and dry. You may also put any needed disposable incontinence pads over the draw sheet. Products used for incontinence are discussed in Chapter 18.

Continue with the top sheet:

9. Place the top sheet on the bed. The wide hem should be even with the head of the mattress, with the seam on the outside. When you fold the hem over, the smooth side will be next to the resident's skin, preventing irritation from any rough edges. The excess sheet will be over the foot of the bed.

10. Open the sheet from the fold so that the sheet covers the entire mattress and hangs evenly on both sides.

11. Place the spread on top of the sheet in the same manner. Make sure the sheet does not hang below the spread on the sides.

12. Tuck in the sheet and spread at the foot, making a mitered corner on the bottom end (Step 8c above).

13. Smooth the sheet and spread from the bottom to the top of the bed, and fold down the top hem of the sheet over the spread.

14. Move to the other side of the bed and finish in the same way, starting with the bottom sheet and finishing with the top sheet and spread. Pull the bottom sheet tight before each tuck to remove wrinkles. (Tuck in the draw sheet tightly if used.)

15. Place a clean case on the pillow: Hold the center of the closed end of the pillow case with your hand and turn it inside out over your hand; then grab the pillow with your hand inside the pillowcase and slide the case over the pillow. Make sure the corners of the pillow fit into the corners of the case. Place the pillow(s) at the head of the bed, and fold the spread over them.

16. Put the blanket at the foot of the bed or in the closet if a resident prefers.

17. Return the bed to low position.

PROCEDURE 14-8 – MAKING AN OCCUPIED BED

1. Lower the head of the bed, and remove the pillow from under the resident's head. (Do this only if the resident is comfortable in a completely flat position.)

2. Remove the spread and any blankets, and place them folded on the chair.

3. Loosen the top and bottom sheets from under the mattress. **Note:** *Side rails may be used for support in moving. If there is any risk that the resident could be injured by hitting the side rail, do not use it. Have another nurse assistant on the opposite side to support the resident if there is any risk of injury; make sure this person is ready to help before you begin.*

4. Help the resident roll over on their side toward you. Raise the side rail and ask them to hold onto it for support. Go to the other side of the bed. Be sure the resident stays covered throughout the procedure.

5. Check for any belongings in the bed.

6. Roll lengthwise (top to bottom) the bottom soiled sheet from the side of the mattress to the center of the bed close to the resident's body. (If the linen is wet or very damp, place a barrier like a plastic-covered padding over the sheet.) Change the mattress pad if it is soiled or scheduled for changing.

7.　If you are using a fitted sheet (shaped to the mattress by elastic edging), follow these steps: Starting at the top corner of the mattress, wrap the edge of the mattress with the corner of the sheet; then go to the bottom of the bed on the same side and wrap the edge. Be sure half the mattress is covered and the sheet is tucked close to the resident.

8.　If you are using a draw sheet follow these steps: Place it in the center of the bed so it covers the middle part of the bed and is tucked close to the resident. Tuck in the draw sheet on the side you are working. A draw sheet is often used for residents needing help with moving and positioning, or sometimes to keep bottom sheets clean and dry. You may also put any needed disposable incontinence pads over the draw sheet. **Note:** *Side rails may be used for support in moving. If there is any risk that the resident could be injured by hitting the side rail, do not use it. Have another nurse assistant on the opposite side to support the resident if there is any risk of injury; make sure this person is ready to help before you begin.*

9.　If you are using a flat sheet follow these steps:

　　a.　Unfold the bottom sheet lengthwise, centered on the bed. Do not shake the linen while unfolding. (Shaking the linen raises dust and organisms.) Be sure the hem seams face the mattress. (This prevents any rough edges from touching the resident.)

　　b.　Slide the sheet so that the hem is even with the foot of the mattress. Be sure to keep the fold in the exact center of the bed from head to foot. (You want the extra length of sheet at the top so that you can tuck it under the mattress.)

　　c.　Open the sheet and fan-fold it lengthwise so that one half of the sheet is next to the rolled dirty sheet.

　　d.　Tuck the top hem in tightly under the mattress at the head of the bed by lifting the mattress edge and sliding the sheet under it. Make a mitered corner:

　　　　i.　Face the side of the bed.

　　　　ii.　With one hand, pick up the top of the sheet hanging down the side of the bed, and lay it on top of the bed so it looks like a triangle.

　　　　iii.　Tuck the remaining sheet under the mattress.

　　　　iv.　Drop the section of sheet that is lying on top of the bed over the side of the bed, and tuck it in.

　　e.　Tuck the remaining sheet under the mattress neatly, starting with the mitered corner down to the foot of the mattress.

　　f.　If you are using a draw sheet, place it in the center of the bed so it covers the middle part of the bed. Fan-fold the excess and tuck it in with the sheet. Tuck in the draw sheet. A draw sheet is often used for residents needing help with moving and positioning, or sometimes to keep bottom sheets clean and dry.

Continue with the next steps:

10.　Flatten the rolled or fan-folded sheets and help the resident roll over the linen toward you, using the procedure for turning them (see Chapter 15, Moving and Positioning). Don't forget first to tell the resident that the roll of linen is behind them. **Note:** *Side rails may be used for support in moving. If there is any risk that the resident could be injured by the use of the rail, do not use it. Put up the side rail and ask the resident to hold onto it for support.*

11.　Go to the opposite side of the bed, lower the side rail, and remove the dirty bottom sheet. **Note:** *Never leave the resident unattended to take away dirty laundry. Put the dirty sheets in the laundry bag (if it is in the room) or at the bottom of the bed between the mattress and footboard.*

12.　Pull the clean linen toward you until it is completely unfolded, and tuck the sheets in tightly the same way as you did on the other side. Tuck in the draw sheet if used.

13.　Help the resident roll back to the center of the bed.

14.　Place the top sheet on the bed over the sheet covering the resident. Open the sheet from the fold so that the sheet hangs evenly on each side of the bed. The wide hem should be at the top with the seam on the outside. When you fold the hem over, the smooth side will be next to the resident's skin, preventing any rough edges from touching them. The excess sheet is over the foot of the bed.

15.　Ask the resident to hold onto the clean sheet, then carefully remove the dirty top sheet by placing your hand under the clean top sheet and rolling the dirty sheet down toward the foot of the bed. Remove it and put it with the other dirty linen.

16　Place the spread on top of the sheet in the same way you did the top sheet. Make sure the sheet does not hang below the spread on the sides.

17.   Tuck in the sheet and spread at the foot of the bed, and make a mitered corner at the bottom ends:
   - a.   Face the side of the bed.
   - b.   With one hand, pick up the top sheet hanging down the side of the bed, and lay it on top of the bed so it looks like a triangle.
   - c.   Tuck the remaining sheet under the mattress.
   - d.   Drop the sheet lying on top of the bed over the side of the bed, and tuck it in.
18.   Smooth the sheet and spread from the bottom to the top of the bed, and fold down the top hem of the sheet over the top of the spread. Be sure the top linens are not so tight that they are pressing on the resident's feet. To be sure, make a toe pleat. This is done by pulling the top linen up to form a pleat.
19.   Remove the dirty pillowcase, and put a clean case on the pillow. Hold the center of the closed end of the pillow case with your hand, turn it inside out over your hand, and then grab the pillow with the hand inside the pillow case and slide the case over the pillow. Make sure the corners of the pillow fit into the corners of the case. Put the pillow under the resident's head.

PROCEDURE 15-1 – MOVING UP IN BED WHEN A RESIDENT CAN HELP
1.   Put the head of the bed flat if the resident can tolerate it. Move the pillows against the headboard.
2.   Help the resident bend their knees up and place their feet flat on the bed. Place one arm under the resident's upper back behind the shoulders and the other under their upper thighs.
3.   On the count of three, have the resident push down with their feet and lift up their buttocks (bridging) while you help move them toward the head of the bed. **Note:** *You may also try having the resident help by using the side rails.*

PROCEDURE 15-2 – MOVING UP IN BED WHEN A RESIDENT IS UNABLE TO HELP
1.   Call another staff person to assist you.
2.   Put the head of the bed flat if the resident can tolerate it. Remove the pillow and place it against the headboard.
3.   Help the resident to cross their hands over their chest.
4.   Roll the draw sheet up from the side toward the resident until you and your helper both have a tight grip on it with both hands. Keep your palms up if that gives you more strength for moving. **Note:** *You can put one knee on the bed to get as close to the resident as possible.*
5.   Count aloud to 3, and you and your helper lift the resident up to the head of the bed, using good body mechanics. You can do this in stages until the resident is in position. **Note:** *If the resident is able, ask them to lift their head off the bed during the move.*
6.   Unroll the draw sheet and tuck it in.

PROCEDURE 15-3 – MOVING TO THE SIDE OF THE BED WHEN A RESIDENT CAN HELP
1.   Stand on the side to which you plan to move the resident.
2.   Help the resident bend their knees up and place their feet on the bed.
3.   Help the resident to bridge (lift up their buttocks), and move their buttocks to the side of the bed.
4.   Help the resident move their legs over, and then their head and upper body, by sliding your arms under them and gliding them toward you if they need help.
5.   You can do this in stages to reach the desired position.

PROCEDURE 15-4 – MOVING TO THE SIDE OF THE BED WHEN A RESIDENT IS UNABLE TO HELP
1.   Stand on the side to which you plan to move the resident.
2.   Ask the resident to fold their arms across their chest or do this for them if needed.
3.   Slide both your hands under the resident's head, neck, and shoulders and glide them toward you on your arms.
4.   Slide your arms under the residents' hips and glide them toward you.
5.   Slide your arms under their legs and glide them toward you.

PROCEDURE 15-5 – MOVING A RESIDENT TO THE SIDE OF THE BED USING A DRAW SHEET

1. _____ Call another staff person to help you.
2. _____ Help the resident place their arms across their chest.
3. _____ Both you and your helper roll up the draw sheet from the sides toward the resident until you both have a good tight grip with both hands. **Note:** *The staff person who is moving the resident away may want to put one knee on the edge of the bed to prevent injury caused by reaching too far. This person also leads the count because they have the heaviest part of the move.*
4. _____ Count aloud to 3, and on 3 you both lift the resident to the side of the bed. You can do this in stages until the desired position is reached.
5. _____ Unroll the draw sheet and tuck it in.

PROCEDURE 15-6 – TURNING A RESIDENT FROM SUPINE TO SIDE-LYING FOR PERSONAL CARE

1. _____ Help the resident bend their knees up one at a time and place their feet flat on the bed.
2. _____ Place one hand on the resident's shoulder farther away from you and the other hand on the hip farther from you.
3. _____ On the count of 3, help the resident roll toward you. Continue personal care.
Note: *Some residents may be more comfortable guiding the turn by holding onto the side rails.*

PROCEDURE 15-7 – MOVING THE RESIDENT FROM SUPINE POSITION TO SITTING

1. _____ Help the resident roll onto their side facing you, or elevate the head of the bed.
2. _____ Reach under the resident's head and put your hand under their shoulder (using your arm closer to the head of the bed). The resident's head should be supported by and resting on your forearm.
3. _____ With your other hand, reach over and behind the resident's knee farther from you.
4. _____ Using your legs and arms to do the lifting, bring the resident's head and trunk up as you swing their legs down to the sitting position. Hold the resident's legs, letting their knees rest in the crook of your elbow. **Note:** *Your arm behind the resident's head and body must stay in contact with the resident once they are sitting up to prevent them from falling backward. Remember to stay directly in front of the resident so you can block them with your body if needed for safety.*
   Note: *If you need a second staff person to help you assist the resident to sit up, both of you stand on the same side. One of you lifts the resident's head and body, while the other lifts their legs.*
5. _____ Help the resident get comfortable in the sitting position.

Another option is to:
1. _____ Help the resident roll onto their side facing you, or elevate the head of the bed.
2. _____ Slide their feet over edge of the bed.
3. _____ Reach under the resident's head and put your hand under their shoulder (using your arm closer to the head of the bed). The resident's head should be supported by and resting on your forearm.
4. _____ Place your other hand on the resident's hip. As you help the resident sit up, place gentle but firm pressure on their hip (using leverage) and help raise the resident's head to a sitting position. **Note:** *Your arm behind the resident's head and body must stay in contact with the resident once they are sitting up to prevent them from falling backward. Remember to stay directly in front of the resident so you can block them with your body if needed for safety.*

PROCEDURE 15-8 – MOVING THE RESIDENT FROM SITTING TO SUPINE POSITION

Note: *Before moving a resident from sitting to the supine position, be sure they are centered in the bed with the backs of their knees against the mattress. Help them push down on the floor with their feet and down on the bed with their hands to move their body back onto the bed in a sitting position.*
1. _____ Place one hand behind the resident's shoulder, and let their head and neck rest on your forearm. Place your other hand under their knees, and let their legs rest in the crook of your elbow. Position your arms as if you were carrying someone in front of you.
2. _____ Use your legs to lift and breathe out as you help the resident lift their legs up onto the bed. Gently lower their trunk and head onto the bed. **Note:** *You might want to elevate the head of the bed before helping the resident into the supine position. Once they are in bed, you can lower the head of the bed.*

PROCEDURE 15-9 – THE STAND PIVOT TRANSFER

1. _____ Stand in front of the resident.
2. _____ Place one of your legs between the resident's legs and the other close to the target you are moving toward, such as a chair. (This gives you better control over the speed and the direction of the movement.)
3. _____ Hold onto the guard belt at the resident's back, slightly to either side. If you are not using a guard belt, put your arms around the resident's waist.
4. _____ Ask or help the resident to push down on the bed with their hands, lean forward, and stand up. If they are not able to do this, you can have them hold your waist during the transfer. Do not let the resident hold you around your neck, which could injure you.
5. _____ On the count of 3 help the resident stand by leaning your body back and up, thereby bringing the resident's body forward. Ask them to lean forward and stand up.
6. _____ Once the resident is standing, keep your back neutral and body facing forward, and pivot (turn on your feet or take small steps) to turn them until the backs of their knees are against the chair.
7. _____ Ask the resident to reach back for the arm of the chair with one or both hands if possible.
8. _____ Help the resident bend their knees and sit.
9. _____ Once the resident is sitting, ask or help them to push back in the chair by pushing down with their feet on the floor and their arms on the armrests.

PROCEDURE 15-10 –ASSISTED TRANSFER WITH AN ASSISTIVE DEVICE (ONE PERSON)

1. _____ Once the resident is sitting on the side of the bed without difficulty, place the assistive device in their hand (cane) or in front of them (walker).
2. _____ Stand to the side of the resident on the side opposite the device.
3. _____ Ask or help the resident to push down on the bed with their hands and stand on the count of 3. You can help them by pulling up and forward on the back of the guard belt with one hand while pushing down on the walker or cane to keep it stable while the resident stands. Encourage a resident using a walker to stand before grabbing onto the assistive device.
4. _____ For residents using a walker, after they are standing, help them put both hands on the walker. **Note:** _Have the resident stand for a few minutes before trying to move, especially if they are dizzy._
5. _____ Help the resident move toward the chair. Guide them with statements like these: "Turn, turn, take a step toward me, now back up."
6. _____ Help the resident back up to the chair. Ask if they can feel the chair against the back of their legs. Explain that they should not sit until they feel this.
7. _____ When the resident is in front of the chair, ask him them to reach back and put one hand on the armrest.
8. _____ Help the resident reach back with the other hand for the arm of the chair and slowly sit down.

PROCEDURE 15-11 – TRANSFERRING A RESIDENT FROM A CHAIR TO A BED, COMMODE, OR TOILET

1. _____ Position the chair with the resident's stronger side closer to the bed, commode, or toilet.
2. _____ If the resident is in a wheelchair, ask them to move their feet off the footrests. Raise up the footrests.
3. _____ Ask the resident to slide forward to the edge of the chair. This is often difficult, and the resident may need help.
4. _____ Use either the stand pivot or assistive device transfer procedure in reverse to move the resident from the chair and into bed.

PROCEDURE 15-12 – MOVING A RESIDENT WITH A MECHANICAL LIFT

1. _____ Adjust the head of the bed as flat as possible if the resident can tolerate it. To put the sling under the resident, first turn the resident toward you. Help the resident move toward you while your helper on the other side of the bed pushes the fan-folded sling under the resident as far as possible. Then help the resident back and toward the other side and pull the sling under them. **Note:** _The sling should be placed from under the resident's shoulders to the back of the knees. Have the same amount of sling material on both sides of the resident so that the resident is centered._
2. _____ Place the lift frame facing the bed with its legs under the bed. Lock the wheels on the base.
3. _____ Elevate the head of the bed so the resident is partially sitting up.
4. _____ Attach the sling to the lift following the manufacturer's directions.

5.   Ask the resident to cross their arms over their chest before operating the lift. **Note:** *If a resident cannot keep their hands in their lap or across their chest, try having them hold onto an object on their lap.*

6.   Follow the manufacturer's directions to raise the resident up to a sitting position with the lift. While you operate the lift, your helper should help you guide the resident. **Note** *Repeatedly ask the resident if they are OK. Reassure the resident because this can be a frightening experience, especially the first time.*

Once the resident is sitting, keep raising the lift until they are 6 to 12 inches over the bed and chair height.

7.   Unlock the swivel, if the lift has one, or use the steering handle to move the resident directly over the chair. You may need to guide the resident's legs.

8.   Tell the resident that you are now going to lower them slowly into the chair. Your helper guides the resident into the chair by moving the sling. Press the release button to slowly lower them down.

9.   Once the resident is securely in the chair, unhook the sling and remove the lift frame.

10.   Position the resident in the chair, leaving the sling under them (unless the sling is removable) until it is time to return to bed. Pull the metal bars of the sling out so that the resident does not lean against or sit on them.

PROCEDURE 15-13 – MOVING A RESIDENT UP IN A CHAIR

Note: *These steps are for moving a resident up in the chair after a transfer procedure to the chair. You need a helper for this procedure.*

1.   Place the guard belt on the resident.

2.   Standing on both sides of the resident, each of you grasps the guard belt with one hand and and puts the other hand under the resident's knees. Ask the resident to cross their arms in front of their chest).

3.   On the count of 3, breathe out and lift the resident back in the chair. Be sure to use good body mechanics.

PROCEDURE 15-14 – RETURNING A RESIDENT TO BED USING A MECHANICAL LIFT

1.   Position the lift facing the chair.

2.   Insert the metal bars into the sling sides.

3.   Hook the chains into the sling holes.

4.   Crank (or raise) the resident up with the lift. Your helper guides the resident by holding the sling.

5.   Swing the frame of the lift over the bed and slowly lower the resident down onto the bed.

6.   Unless the resident will spend only a short time in bed, roll them from side to side to remove the sling. (The sling could cause skin irritation if left under the resident.)

7.   Position the resident as preferred.

PROCEDURE 15-15 – POSITIONING A RESIDENT ON THEIR BACK

1.   First move the resident's trunk and lower body so that their spine is in a neutral position. Do the positioning from the top of the body to the bottom.

2.   Position the resident's head and neck: Place a pillow under the resident's head and neck extending to the top of their shoulders. Do not elevate their head too high. Keep it as close to even with the chest as possible or as is comfortable.

3.   Position the resident's arms. The backs of the shoulders and elbows are common places for pressure ulcers in residents who cannot change positions by themselves. Vary their arm positions to prevent this. Keep their arms straight and resting on the mattress away from their sides, or bend their arms slightly at the elbow with a pillow between the inner arm and their side so that their arm rests on the pillow and their hand on top of the abdomen. Always support the arms in two places when moving them, and move them gently.

4.   Position the resident's legs: The sides of the hips, the buttocks, the sacrum and coccyx (the tip of the spine at the buttocks, or "tail bone"), and the backs of the heels are common places for pressure ulcers. Position the resident's legs straight and slightly apart. Always support the legs in 2 places when moving them, and move them gently. For those residents who tend to keep their legs tightly together or crossed, you may place a pillow between the resident's legs.

Note: *If a resident has ulcers on the sides of the hips, place a towel roll along the hip between the hip and the mattress on the affected side.*

If a resident has redness or ulcers under their heels, support their legs with a pillow lengthwise to raise their heels from the bed, or put a towel roll under their legs just above the heels.

Note: *Support casts, splints, or swollen arms or legs by placing them on a pillow lengthwise to support the hand or foot higher than the rest of their arm or leg.*

PROCEDURE 15-16 – POSITIONING A RESIDENT ON THEIR SIDE (SIDE-LYING POSITION)

1. ____ Stand on the side to which the resident will be turning.
2. ____ Help the resident to bend their knees up.
3. ____ Place one hand on the resident's shoulder farther from you and the other on the hip farther from you. On the count of 3, help the resident roll toward you. Position the resident comfortably with proper body alignment.
4. ____ Position the resident's head and neck. Place the pillow under their head so that their top ear is almost level with their top shoulder.
5. ____ Fold a pillow lengthwise and place it behind the resident's back. Gently push the top edge of the pillow under their side and hip.
6. ____ Position the resident's arms. Gently pull the bottom arm out from under the resident's body if it is not already in front of the body. Place a pillow diagonally under the top arm between the arm and the resident's side. Bend the top arm or the elbow and shoulder to rest the arm on the pillow.
7. ____ Position the resident's legs. Bend the top hip up and rotate it slightly forward. Place a pillow lengthwise between the resident's knees to separate their legs down to their ankles.

Note: *Depending on the resident's condition, you can modify any of these positions to prevent pressure ulcers and make the resident comfortable.*

PROCEDURE 16-1 – COMPLETE BED BATH

Note: *Before beginning the bath, remove the resident's blanket and bedspread and put them on a clean surface. Put a bath blanket over the top sheet and then pull down the top sheet to the foot of the bed, leaving the bath blanket covering the resident. Expose only the part of the resident's body you are washing. This gives the person privacy and prevents them from becoming cold. Remove their clothing also under the bath blanket. The best position for the resident is flat in bed, if they can tolerate it. Fill the water basin halfway with water that is warm to your touch. Test the water with your bare hand– not with gloves on. The water temperature should be 98.6 F to 103 F. You can use a thermometer if one is available, or test the water temperature with the inside of your wrist, and then have the resident feel the water to be sure it is comfortable. Wash, rinse, dry, and inspect each body part. Be gentle. Start by making a bath mitt.*

Making a Bath Mitt: Make a bath mitt with the washcloth. The mitt provides a soft surface for the person's skin and is easier to use than an unfolded washcloth. The edges of an unfolded washcloth may get cold and make the resident uncomfortable.

1. ____ After wringing out the wet washcloth, put your hand in the center of the washcloth.
2. ____ Fold the side of the washcloth over from your little finger, and hold the fold with your thumb.
3. ____ Fold the remaining cloth over and hold it firmly with your thumb.
4. ____ Fold the top edge of the cloth down and tuck it into your palm. Hold it with your thumb.
5. ____ The mitt is now ready to use. Rinse the cloth and refold the mitt as needed during the bath.

Giving a Complete Bed Bath

1. ____ Begin with the resident's eyes, using only water–no soap. Start with the eye that is farther from you. With one corner of the washcloth, wash from the inner corner of the eye outward toward the ear. Clean away any crusting that may be stuck to the lower part of the eye. Use another corner of the washcloth to wash the near eye. Be sure to move the washcloth from the inner corner of the eye outward.
2. ____ Wash the resident's face. Some residents prefer not to use soap on their face. If so, use water only. Rinse, dry, and inspect the area. **Note:** *To wash with soap, wet the washcloth and apply a small amount of soap on it. Be sure to rinse the soap off. When you dry the resident's skin, pat it dry, being careful not to rub too hard.*
3. ____ Wash the resident's ears and neck. Rinse, dry, and inspect the area. **Note:** *When washing the resident's ears, wash behind the ear as well as inside. Wring out the wash cloth so that excess water does not enter the ear canal.*
4. ____ Wash the arms, underarm areas, and hands. Expose only the areas to be washed. Use a bath blanket to cover the resident. Use soap sparingly. (Remember: soap dries the skin.) Wash the side away from you first, then the side near you, so that you are moving from a clean area to a dirty area, unless you feel you have to stretch too far and might injure yourself. (If so, wash one side of the resident's body, then move to the other side and wash it.) Rinse, dry, and inspect the area.
5. ____ Fold the bath blanket down and cover the resident's chest with a towel. Wash the chest and abdomen down as far as the pubic area. Rinse, dry, and inspect the area. Pay particular attention to the skin under a female resident's breasts and or any skin folds on the chest and abdomen. These are common areas for skin irritation and breakdowns. Note any redness, odor, or skin breakdown. Cover the chest with the bath blanket.

6.   Expose one leg, thigh, and foot. Cover the exposed leg with a towel. Wash the legs and feet. Don't forget to wash between the toes. Rinse, dry, and inspect the area. Check between the toes for any redness, irritation, or cracking of the skin. Note any swelling of the feet and legs. **Note:** *Change the water at this time or at any time during the bath if the water gets too cold, soapy, or dirty. (Using the same water after foot washing could potentially spread a foot fungus.) Cover up the resident before leaving to change the water.*

Cover up the resident before leaving to change the water.

7.   Help the resident to turn to one side (see procedures for moving residents in Chapter 16). Keep the resident covered with a bath blanket.

8.   Expose the resident's back and buttocks. Wash the resident's back and buttocks. Rinse, dry, and inspect the area.

9.   Give the resident a back rub. Rub a small amount of lotion into your palms. Starting at the resident's lower back, gently move your hands up toward the shoulders, then downward to the lower back. Give the back rub for at least 3 minutes. Back rubs are comforting and relaxing and stimulate circulation, helping prevent skin breakdown. **Note:** *You may also give a back rub on request or as part of p.m. care.*

10.   Help the resident move back onto their back.

11.   Give perineal care (wash the genital and anal area of the body), as described below. **Note:** *After the back rub and before perineal care, put a plastic-covered pad under the resident to absorb water used to wash the perineal area, and put on a new pair of gloves. You can also use a bedpan for this. The bedpan allows a good view of the perineal area because it raises the resident's pelvis and lets you use more water for washing and rinsing. Since it might be uncomfortable for a resident, ask first. Sometimes you can use a fracture pan or a folded towel under the buttocks to raise the pelvis. Remember these guidelines:*
    - *Always change the water before perineal care.*
    - *Always change the washcloth and towel.*
    - *Always wear gloves when giving perineal care.*

    Note: *Perineal care is described here as part of a complete bed bath. If you do it separately, perform preparation and completion steps before and after the perineal care.*

12.   Help the resident get dressed.

Perineal Care for Female Residents

1.   Help the resident onto the bedpan or pad.

2.   Put on gloves.

3.   Drape the resident by folding back the bath blanket to expose only her legs and perineal area. Ask the resident to bend her knees.

4.   Wash the pubic area first. Separate the labia and wash downward on each side of the labia using different corners of the washcloth. Wash downward in the middle over the urethra and vaginal openings. Always wash downward toward the anus to prevent the spread of infection.

5.   If you used a bedpan, help the resident off the bedpan onto her side. Wash the anal area, moving up toward the back.

6.   Rinse, dry, and inspect the perineal area and then the anal area. Check for any redness, swelling, drainage, odor, or area of irritation.

Perineal Care for Male Residents

1.   Put on gloves.

2.   Drape the resident to expose only his legs and perineal area by folding back the bath blanket.

3.   Wash the penis from the urethral opening or tip of the penis toward the base of the penis, and then wash the scrotum. Take care to wash, rinse, and dry between any skin folds. Pull back the foreskin on uncircumcised males and clean under it. Return the foreskin. Check for any redness, swelling, or areas of irritation.

4.   Help the resident turn onto his side. Wash, rinse, and dry the anal area well, moving upward toward the back.

PROCEDURE 16-2 – TUB BATH

1. _____ Assist the resident to the tub room with all supplies. **Note:** *Some facilities may use chairs on wheels that may be taken to the resident's room. If you use this chair to bring the resident to the tub room, make sure that they are properly dressed and draped to protect their privacy and use the safety straps if needed and available.*
2. _____ Help the resident sit on the chair. Fill the tub halfway with warm water.
3. _____ Remember, always turn the hot water off first. **Note:** *The tub water should be in the range of 98.6 F to 103 F. Use a thermometer if available, or test the water temperature with the inside of your wrist, and then have the resident feel it with their hand or foot. The resident's doctor may order special medication to be added to the bath water, such as bran, oatmeal, starch, sodium bicarbonate, Epsom salts, pine products, sulfa, potassium permanganate, or salt. Always check with the charge nurse about the proper use of any of these substances.*
4. _____ Help the resident remove their clothing.
5. _____ Check that the bath mat is in place. Help the resident into the tub. **Note:** *Never leave the resident alone while bathing in a tub. Always encourage residents to use safety rails. Be sure to check the water temperature during the tub bath to be sure it has not cooled down. Add hot water as needed.*
6. _____ Help with bathing as needed. (Put gloves on if you will be assisting with perineal care.)
7. _____ Place a clean towel on the seat of the chair.
8. _____ Help the resident out of the tub. Encourage them to use safety rails. Cover them with a bath blanket
9. _____ Help the resident with drying, applying personal hygiene products, and dressing. **Note:** *You may give them a back rub before dressing, if the resident desires.*
10. _____ Help the resident back to their room. Bring any of their personal hygiene products back to their room.

PROCEDURE 16-3 – SHOWER

1. _____ Help the resident to the shower room with all necessary supplies.
2. _____ Help the resident sit on the chair, using safety straps if needed and available.
3. _____ Turn on the shower with warm water. Test the water on the inside of your wrist and have the resident feel it with their hand or foot. Adjust the temperature as needed.
4. _____ Help the resident remove their clothing.
5. _____ Help the resident into the shower. Encourage them to use the safety rails. **Note:** *Most facilities have shower chairs that lock in place. If the resident needs to shower sitting down, be sure the shower chair is locked before they sit down.*
6. _____ Help the resident with showering as needed. (Wear gloves if you help with perineal care.) Encourage the resident to participate in bathing as much as possible. Give help and verbal cueing as needed. Wash from head to toe. Rinse the washcloth as needed. **Note:** *Bathing is a good time to observe the resident's skin for any skin conditions, to conduct range-of-motion exercises, and to engage in conversation with the resident. These acts add restorative care into the resident's daily routine.*
   Note: *If the resident is not shampooing, use a shower cap to prevent their hair from getting wet.*
7. _____ Place a dry towel on the chair outside the shower.
8. _____ Help the resident out of the shower and onto the covered chair. Cover the resident with a bath blanket.
9. _____ Turn off the shower. Turn the hot water off first to prevent a burn.
10. _____ Help the resident dry off, use personal hygiene products, and get dressed. **Note:** *You may give a back rub at this point if desired.*
11. _____ Help the resident back to their room. Bring their personal hygiene products back to the room and put them away.

PROCEDURE 16-4 – WHIRLPOOL BATH

1. _____ Help the resident to the whirlpool room with all supplies.
2. _____ Help the resident sit on a chair.
3. _____ Turn on the water in the whirlpool following the facility's procedure. The water temperature should be 98.6 F to 103 F. Test the water temperature on the inside of your wrist, and have the resident feel it with their hand or foot. Adjust the temperature as needed.
4. _____ Help the resident remove their clothing.
5. _____ Help the resident into the whirlpool bath. Encourage use of safety rails. **Note:** *Follow the manufacturer's and facility's guidelines. If you use a mechanical lift, be sure you know how to use it properly.*

6.   Help the resident bathe. Encourage the resident to participate in bathing as much as possible. Give help and verbal cueing as needed. Wash from head to toe. Rinse the wash cloth as needed. Wear gloves if you help with perineal care. Never leave the resident unattended. **Note:** *If the resident has a wound dressing, ask the nurse to remove it before the bath and apply a clean one afterward. If the doctor has ordered an* **antiseptic** *solution in the whirlpool bath, the nurse will add the solution or give you specific instructions.*

7.   Place a dry towel on the chair.

8.   Help the resident out of the whirlpool bath and onto the covered chair. Encourage them to use the safety rails. Cover them with a bath blanket.

9.   Help the resident dry off, apply personal hygiene products, and get dressed. **Note:** *You may give them a back rub at this point if desired.*

10.   Help the resident back to their room.

PROCEDURE 16-5 – SHAMPOOING AND CONDITIONING

1.   Help the resident into a chair.

2.   Comb or brush out any tangles before shampooing.

3.   Turn on the water to a warm temperature, no more than 103° F. Test the water temperature on the inside of your wrist, and have the resident feel it with their hand.

4.   Help the resident take off their clothes for showering or tub bathing. Wash the resident's hair as the resident prefers (some residents want it done first, and some last). If a resident is shampooing at the sink, put the back of the chair against the front of the sink. Pad the rim of the sink with a towel. Position the resident for the method you are using: upright in a shower chair, flat in bed with pillows placed under their shoulders, or tilted in shampoo chair. Protect their clothes with a towel draped over the shoulders. If you are shampooing in bed, you need a shampoo trough, basin, or pail, and a waterproof bed protector.

5.   Wet the hair entirely. Place a face cloth over the resident's eyes to prevent shampoo from getting into the resident's eyes.

6.   Pour a small amount of shampoo into your palm and apply it to the resident's wet hair. Massage the shampoo gently throughout hair and scalp.

7.   Rinse the hair well with warm water.

8.   Apply conditioner, if used.

9.   Rinse the hair well with warm water.

10.   Help the resident out of the shower or tub into the chair. Cover them with a bath blanket. Wrap a towel around their hair. Help them dry off and get dressed. If the resident is in bed, help them wipe their face with the towel used to protect their eyes. Remove the trough or basin from beneath the resident's head. Remove the waterproof sheet from under their head and shoulders. Change the linen as necessary. Position the resident with the head of the bed up.

11.   Dry their hair thoroughly and quickly to prevent chilling. Use a hair dryer on a low setting if available.

12.   Style the resident's hair as they like it. Check for any flaking, reddened areas, or other scalp problems. **Note:** *Some residents use special shampoos or conditioners, often with medicine the doctor orders for a specific condition. Ask the nurse for instructions and read the labels carefully before using them.*

13.   Help the resident back to their room.

PROCEDURE 16-6 – BRUSHING AND FLOSSING

Note: *You can help residents with brushing and flossing at the bedside table or the resident's sink, as they prefer.*

1.   Apply a small amount of toothpaste to the wet toothbrush and set it aside. Mix water and mouthwash in a cup. A solution of half water, half mouthwash is best. Set this aside. Mouthwash is strong and could be harmful to sensitive gums.

2.   Break off or least 18 inches of floss. Set this aside.

3.   Put on gloves. **Note:** *If you know that the resident's gums bleed, talk with the charge nurse about other personal protective equipment you may need, like protective eye wear and face mask.*

4.   Put a towel over the resident's chest to protect their clothing.

5.   Give the resident a small amount of mouthwash solution to swish around in their mouth to rinse it. Place the emesis basin under the resident's chin so they can spit out the solution.

6.   Brush the resident's upper teeth and gums first, moving the brush from the gums to the teeth downward. Then brush the lower teeth and gums moving again from the gums to the teeth upward. Be sure to brush the back of the teeth. Inspect the teeth and gums while brushing.

7.   Brush the tongue gently.
8.   Help the resident rinse their mouth with a little mouthwash solution.
9.   Wrap the ends of the floss around your middle fingers of each hand to get a good grip. Gently insert the floss between each tooth and the next. Move the floss to the gum line and down between the teeth. Wrap the floss around your fingertips to keep using a clean section as you move from tooth to tooth.
10.   Have the resident rinse their mouth thoroughly.
11.   Dry any solution around the resident's mouth or chin.

PROCEDURE 16-7 – CARING FOR DENTURES

1.   Put on gloves.
2.   Ask the resident to remove their dentures and place them in the denture cup. If the resident cannot remove their own dentures, follow these steps.
     a.   Place a towel over the resident's chest.
     b.   Rinse the resident's mouth with mouthwash solution to moisten it. Ask them to swish the solution around, and put the emesis basin under their chin so the resident can spit out the solution.
     c.   Remove the upper denture using a paper towel for a better grip. Loosen the denture by gently rocking it back and forth to help break the seal. Put it in the denture cup.
     d.   Remove lower denture using a paper towel for better grip. Loosen it by gently rocking it back and forth. Put it in the denture cup.
3.   Rinse the resident's mouth with mouthwash solution.
4.   If the resident cannot rinse, use a swab moistened with water and mouthwash to clean the whole mouth, including the tongue and gums.
5.   Explain that you will clean the dentures and then return them.
6.   Take the denture cup with dentures, toothbrush, and toothpaste to the resident's bathroom.
7.   Put toothpaste on the toothbrush.
8.   Turn on cool water (hot water can damage dentures), put a small towel or face cloth on the bottom of the sink, and fill the sink halfway. (This helps prevent dentures from breaking if they slip from your hands.)
9.   Hold the dentures over the sink and brush all surfaces.
10.   Rinse the dentures with cool water.
11.   Return the dentures to the denture cup.
12.   If the resident uses denture adhesive, apply it to the dentures before putting them back in their mouth. If the resident does not want the dentures put back at this time, store them safely. Put them in a denture cup labeled with the resident's name and half filled with cool water.

Note: *Inspect the resident's mouth for bleeding, sores, a dry, coated tongue, and mouth odor. Report any changes to the nurse. If the resident has a partial plate with only a few artificial teeth, handle it the same way as a complete set of dentures. Be careful when you remove the partial plate, which has wires that support the teeth in place.*

PROCEDURE 16-8 – MOUTH CARE FOR COMATOSE RESIDENTS

1.   Gently turn the resident's head toward you and elevate the head of the bed (if they can tolerate it) to prevent aspiration.
2.   Put a towel over the resident's chest to protect their clothing.
3.   Put on gloves.
4.   Gently open the resident's mouth and inspect the mouth, teeth, gums, and tongue for changes or signs of injury: bleeding sores, loose or broken teeth, dry coated tongue, or mouth odor. Using a toothette dipped in mouthwash, clean the inside of the mouth (gums, tongue, teeth, roof of the mouth, and insides of the cheeks). **Note:** *Tap excess mouthwash off the toothette. Excess fluid can drip back into their throat and potentially cause aspiration.*
5.   Using a corner of the towel draped over the resident's chest, dry any solution from around their mouth and chin.
6.   Dispose of toothettes as you use them into the plastic trash bag.
7.   Put protective jelly or lip balm on their lips to moisten them.

PROCEDURE 16-9 – SHAVING A MALE RESIDENT'S FACE

1. _____ Observe the resident's face for any moles, rashes, or cuts. Do not shave those areas, or use extra care.
2. _____ Place a towel over the resident's chest to protect their clothing.
3. _____ Put on gloves.
4. _____ Using a face cloth, wet the entire beard with warm water and apply shaving cream with your hands.
5. _____ When the beard is well lathered and softened, start shaving. Shave in the direction the beard grows. Hold the skin tight and smooth by pulling the skin upward with one hand and shaving with a downward stroke with your other hand. Use short, even strokes. Be particularly careful with the neck, chin, and upper lip. Use upward strokes for the neck, downward and slightly diagonal strokes for the chin, and very short downward strokes above the lip.
6. _____ Rinse the razor in warm water after each stroke.
7. _____ Wash and rinse the resident's face with the washcloth, dry his face, and apply aftershave lotion if he prefers.
8. _____ Give the resident a mirror to look at his face.
9. _____ Remove the towel from the resident's chest.

PROCEDURE 16-10 – SHAVING A FEMALE RESIDENT'S UNDERARMS

1. _____ Put the towel under the resident's shoulder on the side you are working from.
2. _____ Raise the resident's arm up along their ear to expose the underarm.
3. _____ Wash the area with warm water.
4. _____ Lather some soap and apply it over the area to be shaved.
5. _____ Carefully shave the area, moving the razor downward from the arm toward the chest.
6. _____ Rinse the soap away thoroughly and pat the area dry.
7. _____ Move the towel to under the opposite shoulder and repeat the steps above.

PROCEDURE 16-11 – SHAVING A FEMALE RESIDENT'S LEGS

1. _____ Place a towel under the resident's leg to be shaved.
2. _____ Wash the part of the leg to be shaved with warm water.
3. _____ Lather some soap or use shaving cream. Spread it over the entire area to be shaved.
4. _____ Carefully shave the area, moving the razor upward from the ankle to the knee. **Note:** *Ask the resident if she wants the area above her knee shaved.*
5. _____ Be sure to rinse the soap thoroughly and pat the area dry.
6. _____ Move the towel under the other leg and repeat the steps above.

PROCEDURE 16-12 – TRIMMING FACIAL HAIR

1. _____ Using safety scissors, carefully trim the facial hair. Be careful not to trim too close to the skin.
2. _____ Give the resident a mirror to look at her face.

PROCEDURE 16-13 – HAIR CARE

1. _____ Brush hair gently. If the resident's hair is long and tangled, remove tangles first with a comb. Start at the ends and work your way up to the scalp.
2. _____ Gently brush and style the hair to the resident's preference. Use any personal items they may request, such as hair spray, clips, or gel.
3. _____ Give the resident a mirror so they can see their hair.

PROCEDURE 16-14 – CARE OF FINGERNAILS

1. _____ Place the basin of warm water on the over-bed table.
2. _____ Ask the resident to soak their hands in the basin 3-5 minutes.
3. _____ Leaving one hand in the water, wash and rinse the resident's other hand. Dry the hand and place it on a dry towel.
4. _____ Clean under the nails with the orangewood stick.
5. _____ Repeat with the other hand.
6. _____ Inspect the resident's hands for cracks in the skin, unusual spots or discoloration, and rough areas.
7. _____ Trim the resident's fingernails using the nail clipper. Clip nails straight across. Shape and remove any rough edges using an emery board or nail file.
8. _____ Put lotion on the resident's hands and gently massage the hands from fingertips toward the wrists to stimulate circulation.
9. _____ Tell the nurse about any redness, irritation, broken skin, or loose skin.

PROCEDURE 16-15 – CARE OF TOENAILS

1. _____ To give foot care to a resident sitting in a chair, put a towel on the floor and the basin of water on the towel. **Note:** *Foot care can be done while a resident is in bed, usually during a bed bath. Put a towel on the bed and the basin on the towel. Ask the resident to flex their leg and soak one foot at a time.*
2. _____ Help the resident to remove their shoes and socks.
3. _____ Place the resident's feet in the basin of warm water.
4. _____ Soak the feet for 3-5 minutes.
5. _____ Clean under the toenails with the orangewood stick to remove any dirt. Scrub callused areas with a warm wash cloth.
6. _____ Wash, rinse, dry, and inspect the feet thoroughly. Report any redness, irritation, or cracked, broken, loose, dry, or discolored skin. Report any callused areas, corns, or loose or broken nails.
7. _____ Apply lotion to the tops of the feet, soles of the feet, and heels. Do not apply lotion between the toes.
8. _____ Help the resident put on clean stockings or socks and shoes.
9. _____ Tell the charge nurse if the resident needs toenail trimming.

PROCEDURE 16-16 – DRESSING A DEPENDENT RESIDENT

Note: *If a resident has a weak or paralyzed arm or has an IV in one arm, help them to put a shirt or dress sleeve on that arm first. With an IV, move the solution through the sleeve first and hang it on the pole. Gently guide the resident's arm through the sleeve, being careful not to dislodge the IV needle or tube. If the resident has an IV pump, call the nurse for assistance. Use this method also for a weak leg. Dress the weak side first.*

1. _____ Remove the resident's gown or pajamas. **Note:** *For privacy and to prevent chill, remove the top portion of the resident's gown or pajamas first. Help the resident dress on top with clean clothes, and then move to the bottom.*
2. _____ Help the resident put on their undershirt or bra, shirt or blouse, or dress.
3. _____ Help the resident put on underwear, stockings or socks, and pants or a skirt. Depending on the type of garment, follow these steps:
   To put on a garment that opens in the back:
   a. _____ Slide the garment onto the resident's arm and shoulder on the weaker side.
   b. _____ Slide the garment onto the arm and shoulder of the stronger side.
   c. _____ Bring the sides of the garment to the back.
   d. _____ Turn the resident toward you, and bring the side of the garments to the back.
   e. _____ Turn the resident away from you, and bring the other side of the garment to the resident's back.
   f. _____ Fasten the buttons, snaps, ties, or zipper.
   g. _____ Place the resident in the supine position.

To put on a garment that opens in the front:

a. _____ Slide the garment onto the resident's arm and shoulder on the weaker side.

b. _____ Bring the resident to a sitting position, and bring the garment around the back. Lower the resident to the supine position.

c. _____ Slide the garment onto the resident's arm and shoulder on the stronger side.

d. _____ Fasten buttons, snaps, ties, or zipper.

To put on a pullover garment:

a. _____ Place the resident in the supine position.

b. _____ Bring the neck of the garment over the resident's head.

c. _____ Slide the arm and shoulder of the garment onto the resident's weaker side.

d. _____ Raise the resident to a semi-sitting position, bring the garment down over the their shoulder, and slide the arm and shoulder of the garment on the resident's stronger side. **Note:** *If the resident cannot assume a sitting position, turn the resident toward you and pull the garment down on the back. Then turn the resident to the other side, and slide their stronger arm and shoulder into the garment. Pull the garment down in the back.*

e. _____ Fasten the buttons, snaps, ties, or zipper.

To put on pants or slacks:

a. _____ Slide the pants over the resident's feet and up their legs.

b. _____ Ask the resident to raise their hips and buttocks off the bed.

c. _____ Bring the pants up over their buttocks and hips. **Note:** *If the resident cannot raise their buttocks and hips, turn them onto their stronger side. Then pull the pants up over their hips and buttocks on their weaker side. Turn the resident onto the other side and repeat the process.*

d. _____ Fasten the buttons, snaps, ties, or zipper.

4. _____ Help the resident put on socks, shoes, or non-skid slippers before they stand, so that they do not slip on the floor. When you put their shoes on in bed, put a pad on the bed to protect bedding.

5. _____ Help the resident stand so you can smooth out their clothing and fasten and neatly tuck in their shirt or blouse.

6. _____ Help them put on any accessories they want to wear.

7. _____ If a resident has a prosthesis or adaptive equipment (such as eyeglasses, dentures, hearing aid, or an artificial limb), help the resident to put the item on.

8. _____ Collect soiled garments, and place them in a hamper for the laundry according to the facility's procedure.

Note: *Residents are usually helped out of bed after dressing for the day.*

PROCEDURE 16-17 – UNDRESSING A DEPENDENT RESIDENT

Note: *This procedure is easier if the resident is sitting on the side of the bed.*

Note: *If a resident has a weak or paralyzed arm or an IV, remove clothing from other side first and then from the weak side or the side with the IV. If the resident has an IV, carefully guide the tubing and solution through the sleeve as the resident's arm moves.*

1. _____ Help the resident remove upper garments (shirt, dress, blouse, and undergarments).

2. _____ Help the resident put on the top half of their pajamas or nightgown.

3. _____ Help the resident remove their shoes or stockings and pants or skirt.

4. _____ If wearing pajamas, help them put on their bottoms.

5. _____ Help the resident into bed.

PROCEDURE 17-1 – MEASURING HEIGHT AND WEIGHT USING AN UPRIGHT SCALE

1. _____ Determine if the resident can walk to the scale or whether you need to bring a portable scale to their room.
2. _____ Before they step on the scale, adjust the height measurement bar so it is higher than the resident's height.
3. _____ Ask the resident what their height is as a check for accuracy.
4. _____ Clear the scale and make sure it is balanced. It should register 0 when the weights are moved all the way over to the left.
5. _____ Place a paper towel on the scale platform. Ask the resident to remove their shoes. Help them stand on the scale. Make sure they are not holding anything.
6. _____ Have the resident stand up straight, with their arms by their side and their eyes looking forward. Slowly lower the height measurement bar to the top of their head. Record their height in feet and inches.
7. _____ Measure the resident's weight by moving the weights to the right until the balance needle is centered. **Note:** *If the weight is 5 pounds or more different from the previous measurement, weigh the resident again before reporting it to the charge nurse. If the resident is wearing a cast or brace when they are weighed, also report this to the nurse.*
8. _____ Help the resident off the scale.
9. _____ Record the resident's height and weight on the worksheet and report the findings to the charge nurse. Example of charting: Height: 5 feet 6 inches, Weight: 135 lbs

Note: *Your facility may have special scales for weighing residents while they are in a wheelchair or confined to bed. Follow your facility's policy and the manufacturer's instructions for using different scales.*

PROCEDURE 18-1 – HELPING A RESIDENT USE A BEDPAN

1. _____ Put on gloves. **Note:** *If you contaminate your gloves in any way during the procedure, you must change to a new pair of gloves.*
2. _____ Put a pad or cover on the surface where you will put the bedpan after it is used.
3. _____ Fold the bedspread and blanket down to the bottom of the bed, leaving the top sheet in place to cover the resident's lower legs. Help the resident lift their nightgown or remove pajama bottoms or underpants.
4. _____ Put a protective cover under the resident's buttocks to protect the bed linen.
5. _____ Ask the resident to bend both knees and lift their buttocks up while you slide the bedpan underneath them. Adjust it for the resident's comfort. Sometimes using powder or cornstarch on the bedpan prevents the resident's skin from sticking to it when the bedpan is removed. **Note:** *If the resident does not have the strength to lift their buttocks, ask or help them turn onto one side (as described in Chapter 15). Hold the bedpan flush against their buttocks and have the resident turn back onto the bedpan. (You may need help from another nurse assistant.)*
6. _____ Remove your gloves and dispose of them.
7. _____ Cover the resident with the top sheet for privacy.
8. _____ Elevate the head of the bed slowly until the resident is in a sitting position. (Remember: You are trying to create a normal setting.) Ask the resident if they are as comfortable as they can be. Change the position of the bedpan if needed to make them comfortable.
9. _____ Provide toilet paper and position the call light button so the resident can reach it. Tell them to call you when finished. If a resident cannot tell you they are finished, check on them every 5 minutes. Because a bedpan puts pressure on the skin, do not leave a resident on a bedpan longer than needed.

To help a resident from the bedpan:

10. _____ Put on gloves.
11. _____ Lower the head of the bed. Ask the resident to lift their buttocks up while you slide the bedpan out. If needed, help them roll onto one side while you hold the bedpan to prevent a spill. Move the bedpan to the covered surface.
12. _____ If needed, help with wiping the perineal area. Put the used toilet tissue in the bedpan. You may need to wash the perineal area for some residents. (Remember to wash, rinse, and dry thoroughly.) Wash or wipe from front to back. Remove and dispose of the protective pad over the bed linen. **Note:** *Some facilities may have premoistened disposable washcloths for perineal care or use a commercial cleanser that is put in a bottle. You squeeze this solution from the bottle over the perineal area.*
13. _____ Remove your soiled gloves and put on clean gloves.
14. _____ Help the resident wash their hands. **Note:** *If perineal washing was necessary, change the water and use a fresh washcloth and towel for hand washing. Remove your gloves, dispose of them, and put on a new pair before proceeding.*
15. _____ Help the resident get dressed.

16. _____ Put the bedpan cover on the bedpan and dispose of the contents in the resident's toilet. Clean the bedpan and return it to the bedside table. Remove and dispose of the protective pad on which you put the bedpan. **Note:** *Most facilities have a water sprayer attached to the toilet for cleaning bedpans, urinals, etc. You will learn the procedure for emptying and cleaning equipment in your facility. When you clean the equipment, be careful not to splash the contents.*

17. _____ Remove and dispose of your gloves in the disposable trash bag, throw the trash bag away, and wash your hands.

PROCEDURE 18-2 – HELPING A MALE RESIDENT USE A URINAL

1. _____ Put on gloves.**Note:** *If you contaminate your gloves in any way during the procedure, you must change to a new pair of gloves.*

2. _____ Put a pad or cover on the surface where you will put the urinal after use. **Note:** *If the resident can stand beside the bed to use the urinal, help him to stand, and provide privacy. Put the call light button within reach so he can call you when finished; then continue with Steps 6-12.*

If a resident uses the urinal while in bed, follow these steps:

3. _____ Fold the bedspread and blanket down to the bottom of the bed, leaving the top sheet over the resident. Help the resident lower his bottom clothing.

4. _____ Place the urinal between the resident's legs at an angle to avoid urine spillage. Gently place the penis into the urinal.

5. _____ Take off your gloves and put them in a plastic trashbag. Cover the resident with the top sheet and give him the call light. Tell him to call you when he is done. Check in a few minutes if he does not call you.

6. _____ Put on new gloves.

7. _____ When the resident is finished, remove the urinal and place it on the covered surface.

8. _____ If needed, help the resident wipe off excess urine with toilet tissue. Dispose of tissue and your gloves in the plastic trash bag.

9. _____ Put on new gloves.

10. _____ Help the resident wash, rinse, and dry his hands.

11. _____ Empty the urinal, clean it, and replace it in the bedside table. **Note:** *most facilities have a water sprayer attached to the toilet for cleaning bedpans, urinals, etc. You will learn the procedure for emptying and cleaning equipment in your facility. When you clean the equipment, be careful not to splash the contents.*

12. _____ Remove and dispose of your gloves in the disposable trash bag, throw the trash bag away, and wash your hands.

PROCEDURE 18-3 – HELPING A RESIDENT USE A PORTABLE COMMODE

1. _____ Put on gloves. **Note:** *If you contaminate your gloves in any way during the procedure, you must change to a new pair of gloves.*

2. _____ Help the resident out of bed to a standing position (as described in Chapter 15, Moving and Positioning). Help pull down the resident's lower clothing. Help them sit on the commode positioned by the bed. **Note:** *Position the commode so it will not move when you help the resident out of bed. Put the commode against the wall or against the bedside table to keep it from moving.*

3. _____ Provide toilet paper and put the call light button within reach.

4. _____ If the resident needs help with wiping when finished:
   a. _____ Put on gloves.
   b. _____ Help with wiping, and throw the tissue into the commode or plastic trash bag.
   c. _____ Take off your gloves and put them in the plastic trash bag.

5. _____ Help the resident with their clothing and to get back into the bed or chair.

6. _____ Put on new gloves.

7. _____ Help the resident wash, rinse, and dry their hands.

8. _____ Remove the container from the commode and empty its contents into the toilet in the bathroom. **Note:** *Most facilities have a water sprayer attached to the toilet for cleaning bedpans, urinals, etc. You will learn the procedure for emptying and cleaning equipment in your facility. When you clean the equipment, be careful not to splash the contents.*

9. _____ Clean and dry the container and put it back in the commode.

10. _____ Remove and dispose of your gloves in the disposable trash bag, throw the trash bag away, and wash your hands.

PROCEDURE 18-4 – COLLECTING A URINALYSIS SPECIMEN

1. ____ Have the resident void or urinate into a bedpan, urinal (if male), or clean hat in the toilet.
2. ____ Put on gloves. **Note:** *If you contaminate your gloves in any way during the procedure, you must change to a new pair of gloves.*
3. ____ Pour about 60 cc of urine in the specimen container. Discard the urine left over by emptying it into the toilet.
4. ____ Write the resident's name, room number, and date and time you collected the specimen on the container's label.
5. ____ Place the specimen container in a biohazardous plastic bag and close it properly.
6. ____ Remove and dispose of your gloves in the disposable trash bag, throw the trash bag away, and wash your hands.

PROCEDURE 18-5 – COLLECTING A CLEAN-CATCH URINALYSIS SPECIMEN

1. ____ Put on gloves. **Note:** *If you contaminate your gloves in any way during the procedure, you must change to a new pair of gloves.*
2. ____ Clean the urethral opening.
   a. ____ For a female resident, use one wipe to clean one side of the labia, a second wipe to clean the other side of the labia, and a third wipe to clean down the middle. Always clean in single strokes from front to back. Use each wipe only once and then dispose of it.
   b. ____ Clean the penis following the procedure used for perineal care. For an uncircumcised male resident, pull back the foreskin of the penis to clean it.
3. ____ Have the resident begin to urinate and then stop if they can. Do not collect this first urine. **Note:** *If the resident cannot stop the flow of urine, you have to put the container under the stream before they finish to get enough urine.*
4. ____ Hold the specimen container under the urethra, ask the resident to begin voiding again, and collect the remainder of the specimen.
5. ____ Write the resident's name, room number, and the date and time you collected specimen on the specimen container.
6. ____ Place the specimen container in a plastic bag and close it.
7. ____ Remove and dispose of your gloves in the disposable trash bag, throw the trash bag away, and wash your hands after handling each specimen.

PROCEDURE 18-6 – COLLECTING A 24-HOUR URINE SPECIMEN

1. ____ Remind the resident not to throw out any urine. Place a sign in the bathroom to alert other staff or family. (Everyone involved needs to understand that if any urine is lost, the test may need to be restarted.) All urine must be collected in the same container.
2. ____ Always put on gloves before handling specimens.
3. ____ Discard the first voided urine of the day. At this time the collection period of 24 hours begins. (The test would be inaccurate if the first voided urine was not discarded, because it contains urine that collected in the bladder before the starting period.) During the collection period the resident should use a bedpan, commode, urinal, or collection hat on the toilet. Remind the resident to call you each time they urinate so that you can be sure all urine specimens are collected.
4. ____ Remove and dispose of your gloves in the disposable trash bag, throw the trash bag away, and wash your hands after handling each specimen.

When the 24 hours are up:
5. ____ Put on a new pair of gloves.
6. ____ Write the resident's name, room number, and the date and the collection time period on the specimen container.
7. ____ Place the specimen container in a biohazardous plastic bag and close it.
8. ____ Remove and dispose of your gloves in the disposable trash bag, throw the trash bag away, and wash your hands after handling each specimen.

PROCEDURE 18-7 — TESTING URINE FOR GLUCOSE AND KETONES (SUGAR AND ACETONE)

1. _____ Put on gloves. **Note:** *If you contaminate your gloves in any way during the procedure, you must change to a new pair of gloves.*
2. _____ Have the resident void in the bedpan, urinal, or hat on a toilet.
3. _____ Either dip the end of the strip in the fresh urine or pass it through the urine stream.
4. _____ Pull the edge of the strip over the rim of the container you are collecting the urine in to get rid of excess urine.
5. _____ Wait 15 seconds (follow the bottle's directions for the time) and compare the ketone portion of the test strip with the ketone color chart on the test strip bottle. Or the strip may show a + or − symbol.
6. _____ Wait 15 seconds more (follow the bottle's directions for the time) and compare the glucose portion of the test strip with the glucose color chart on the test strip bottle. Or the strip may show a + or − symbol. (The total time for testing for glucose and ketones should not exceed 30 seconds. Ignore any color change after this.) **Note:** *Checking for other substances in the urine, such as blood or protein, is done in a similar way. Check the directions for what time of day to do the test and how long to wait for the result.*
7. _____ Remove and dispose of your gloves in the disposable trash bag, throw the trash bag away, and wash your hands after handling each specimen.

PROCEDURE 18-8 — TESTING A STOOL SPECIMEN FOR OCCULT BLEEDING

1. _____ Put on gloves. **Note:** *If you contaminate your gloves in any way during the procedure, you must change to a new pair of gloves.*
2. _____ After the resident has a bowel movement, use an applicator to obtain a small sample of the fecal material.
3. _____ Put a thin smear of the fecal material on the kit's test slide in the designated area. Some test slides have two sections so that you can test smears from two different areas of the stool.
4. _____ After putting the smear on the slide, wait 3–5 minutes. (This allows the slide to better absorb the fecal matter.)
5. _____ Put two drops of the developer solution on the back of the slide directly behind the stool sample.
6. _____ Read the results in 60 seconds (or follow the directions in the kit). If any blue or blue−green color appears around the edge of the sample, the test is positive for occult bleeding. **Note:** *Testing is often done with 3 consecutive stools because bleeding may occur only at times rather than continuously. Checking three stools at different times can better identify occult bleeding.*
7. _____ Remove and dispose of your gloves in the disposable trash bag, throw the trash bag away, and wash your hands after handling each specimen.

PROCEDURE 19-1 — RANGE-OF-MOTION EXERCISES

Note: *Do each exercise 5-10 times, depending on the resident's comfort level with each extremity.*

The Shoulder
1. _____ Help the resident to lift their arm up toward the head of the bed with the elbow straight (flexion).
2. _____ Bring the arm back down to the bed (extension).
3. _____ Help the resident to lift their arm out to the side with the elbow straight (abduction).
4. _____ Bring the arm back toward the side (adduction).
5. _____ Help the resident lift their arm halfway out to the side. With the elbow bent rotate the arm down (internal rotation) and up (external rotation).

The Elbow
1. _____ Help the resident bend the elbow by bringing the hand toward the upper arm with the palm facing up (flexion).
2. _____ Help the resident straighten the elbow by bringing the hand down toward the bed until the elbow is as straight as possible (extension).
3. _____ Help the resident turn their palm over with the elbow fairly straight and the wrist neutral (pronation).
4. _____ Help the resident turn their palm back up with the elbow fairly straight and the wrist neutral (supination).

The Wrist
1. _____ Help the resident bend their wrist down (flexion).
2. _____ Help the resident bend their wrist back (extension).
3. _____ Help the resident move their hand toward the little finger side of the wrist (ulnar deviation).
4. _____ Help the resident move their hand toward the thumb side of the wrist (radial deviation).

The Hand

1. _____ Bend and straighten each finger at each of the creases (joints of the fingers). Then curl the hand into a fist, and straighten the fingers back out (flexion and extension).
2. _____ Spread the fingers away from each other one at a time (abduction) and then back together one at a time (adduction).
3. _____ Bring each finger across the palm to the thumb and back out (opposition).

The Leg

1. _____ Start with the hip and work your way down to the foot.

The Hip

1. _____ Help the resident bring their leg up toward the chest with the knee bent (flexion).
2. _____ Bring their leg back down toward the bed (extension).
3. _____ Help the resident bring their leg out to the side (abduction).
4. _____ Bring their leg back toward the other leg (adduction).
5. _____ Help the resident bring the leg partly up toward the chest with the knee bent. Now gently turn the leg in (internal rotation) and out (external rotation).

The Knee

1. _____ Help the resident bend the leg up toward the chest slightly. From this position, help them bend the knee (flexion).
2. _____ With the hip in the same position as described above, help the resident straighten the knee (extension).

The Ankle

1. _____ Help the resident bend the foot up toward the head while the knee is held straight (dorsiflexion), and then point the foot downward (plantarflexion).
2. _____ Help the resident turn the bottom of the foot outward (eversion) and then inward (inversion).

The Foot

1. _____ As with the hand, place your fingers around each of the resident's toes and gently bend (flexion) and straighten each toe at each of the joints (extension). You can also bend and straighten all the toes at once.

PROCEDURE 19-2 – ASSISTING WITH WALKING

1. _____ Put the guard belt on the resident.
2. _____ If the resident walks without an assistive device, stand at their side so that you can watch their face as you hold onto the belt from behind. If the resident uses a walker or cane, stand on that side with one hand on the back of the belt and the other on the walker (or cane if the resident needs help with the cane). Most residents who use a cane can hold it by themselves, so you can stand on the other side. Make sure that the resident holds the cane in the correct hand.
3. _____ Walk with the resident. Have them take small steps and slowly progress to larger ones. When walking in hallways, encourage residents not using a walker to use the safety bars for added support. Always stand on their other side so they may use the bars.